A PARENT'S GUIDE

Your Child's
EPILEPSY

Richard E. Appleton MA, FRCP
*Consultant Paediatric Neurologist and Director of the
Roald Dahl EEG Unit, Royal Liverpool Children's
Hospital (Alder Hey), Liverpool*

Brian Chappell BEd
*National Manager, Neuroeducation, Department of
Neurosciences, York District Hospital; former Director of
Information and Training, British Epilepsy Association*

Margaret Beirne ECNE
*Chief Neurophysiology Technician, Roald Dahl EEG Unit,
Royal Liverpool Children's Hospital (Alder Hey),
Liverpool*

CLASS PUBLISHING · LONDON

The rights of Richard E. Appleton, Brian Chappell and Margaret Beirne
to be identified as the authors of this work have been asserted by them in
accordance with the Copyright, Design and Patents Act 1988

The charter for people with epilepsy is the copyright of the British
Epilepsy Association and has been reprinted with their kind permission

Printing history
First published 1997

The authors and publishers welcome feedback from the users of this
book. Please contact the publishers.
**Class Publishing (London) Ltd, Barb House, Barb Mews,
London W6 7PA**
Telephone: 0171 371 2119
Fax: 0171 371 2878 [International +44171]

A CIP catalogue record for this book is available from the British Library

ISBN 1 872362 61 3

Designed by Wendy Bann

Edited and indexed by Susan Bosanko

Cartoons by Jane Taylor

Line illustrations by David Woodroffe

Produced by Landmark Production Consultants Ltd, Princes Risborough

Typesetting by DP Photosetting, Aylesbury, Bucks

Printed and bound in Great Britain by Clays Ltd, St Ives plc

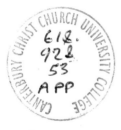

Contents

Acknowledgements

We are grateful to all the people who have helped in the production of this book, and in particular we would like to thank the following people for their contributions and support:

Linda Finnegan for her assistance in the preparation of the manuscript;

Avril Stewart CQSW for all her help and advice;

Hilary Kent, Director of Information and Training at the British Epilepsy Association for her help and advice, and for reviewing the manuscript;

the staff of the British Epilepsy Association National Information Centre for collecting many of the questions for us;

Jill Pooley, former Director of Information and Training at the British Epilepsy Association for reviewing the manuscript;

and last, but certainly not least, the children with epilepsy and their parents who contributed to the section on My Child's Epilepsy, reviewed the manuscript of the book and posed for the cover photograph - many of them asked to remain anonymous, so we are not listing any of their names here, but we are grateful to all of them for their invaluable assistance.

Foreword
by The Lord Hastings

President, British Epilepsy Association 1965–1993; Chairman, Epilepsy Research Foundation 1991–1996

The first thing to strike me about this book is its extreme readability. Technical jargon, which inevitably surrounds the subject of epilepsy and which can bemuse and even frighten the non-professional reader, is rendered easily understandable by the use of plain English.

The second thing which must recommend this book to every parent who has a child with epilepsy is the clearly defined arrangement of the chapters and the format used, that of question and answer. This makes it easy to find the information and advice required on any and every aspect of epilepsy and its consequences, whether medical, social or domestic.

The very comprehensiveness of *Your child's epilepsy* and its essentially practical nature, including glossary and useful organisations, will make it of exceptional value not only to parents and to the children themselves, but also to GPs who will find that a copy in their surgery will be a helpful asset and a time saver.

Hastings

Foreword
by Professor David Chadwick MD, FRCP

Professor of Neurology, The University of Liverpool

Epilepsy is no respecter of age. It most commonly presents in childhood and tends to be seen at its most severe during the childhood years. It remains a uniquely frightening, stigmatising and misunderstood disorder. For all these reasons the impact of epilepsy in a child on all the family members can be enormous.

Many studies have shown the considerable informational needs of people with epilepsy and their carers. While the void that previously existed has been filled with a number of books and by informational material from the epilepsy associations, the needs of parents of children with epilepsy have been somewhat neglected. This book addresses their needs in a very straightforward, user-friendly fashion, with a question and answer format and also contains insights from parents of children with epilepsy that others will find useful.

I am delighted that colleagues from Liverpool have been involved in the development and production of this book. It has been my pleasure to work very closely with Richard Appleton over the last few years and there is no doubt that his impact on the care offered to children with epilepsy within our region has been very considerable. His kindness, understanding and skill is very much reflected in this book which should be of enormous value to any parent reading it.

David Chadwick.

The Charter for People with Epilepsy

The British Epilepsy Association believes that people with epilepsy:

- are individuals and should be respected and treated as such;
- should be offered education and training opportunities in the community to suit their needs and abilities;
- are entitled to employment policies and procedures based on their skills, experience and qualifications;
- sometimes have particular needs which should be met by a system of disability benefits and allowances;
- deserve quality medical care from practitioners who understand epilepsy, on a free and accessible basis;
- have the right to information to help them choose whether or not to undergo any treatment offered;
- should be able to say 'I have epilepsy' without being rejected or labelled by others.

Introduction

To be told that your child has epilepsy can be a shocking or even a traumatic experience for any parent. Faced with this news, most parents are anxious to obtain all the facts and to learn as much about epilepsy as they possibly can. A great deal of information is already available in various formats – medical textbooks, books, leaflets, videos, audiocassettes, even computer packages. There are also various epilepsy associations which can provide help, advice and information. So why, with all this information available, is there a need for another book on the subject?

Above all, we felt that parents of children with epilepsy deserved a book which was written especially for them. To the best of our knowledge *Your Child's Epilepsy – A Parent's Guide* is the first British book about epilepsy specifically written for parents, despite the fact that about 80 parents a day are told that their children have epilepsy. The questions we have answered are real questions which have been asked by many parents of children with epilepsy. We have tried to cover all aspects of epilepsy in children: as well as the obvious medical issues (eg the different types of epilepsy and the different treatments available), there are many questions on the important social issues which relate to children (eg school, other people's attitudes to epilepsy, sports and other recreational activities, and growing up).

What about the other obvious sources of information – for example, the doctors who are looking after your child's

1

epilepsy? Doctors and other health professionals are often seen by the families of people with epilepsy as the 'experts' and certainly they have an important role to play in helping to ensure successful medical treatment. However, it is unfortunate (but understandable) that not every doctor has specialist knowledge about epilepsy and some parents may therefore experience some difficulty in obtaining all the information they would like to have. Fear of 'wasting the doctor's time' may mean that parents are reluctant to ask questions, or to ask for an answer to be explained in more detail, or to ask for information to be repeated (although none of these things are time-wasting). Even when a lot of facts about epilepsy are provided, parents may be unclear as to whether all these facts apply to their own child as each child is different. Some parents may not have their specific questions answered, whatever their source of information.

Medical advances happen all the time and some of these advances will make things easier for children with epilepsy, but we are not yet in sight of a cure or a 'magic' pill which will solve everyone's problems. Certainly a change in society's attitude to epilepsy could – and would – make many people's lives easier. As with so many things in life, it is you and your family who can make the most difference. We hope that this book will provide you with some ideas and help while you are trying to find out more about your child's epilepsy, that you will also find it useful and informative, and that it will answer some, or even most, of the questions that you wanted to ask.

Finally, what are dogs doing in a book about epilepsy? A dog seemed to us to be a suitable 'mascot' for this book, as dogs can have epilepsy and be treated for it too (as can cats, horses and other animals – they all have brains so they can all have epilepsy). Some dogs can even sense when a human is about to have an epileptic seizure. Jane Taylor, our cartoonist, has epilepsy herself and so has been able to add her personal experience to produce her entertaining cartoons.

HOW TO USE THIS BOOK

Because different parents will have different requirements for information about their child's epilepsy, this book has been designed in such a way that you do not have to read it from cover to cover (unless you wish to do so). Instead it can be used selectively to meet your own particular needs. The questions are arranged into chapters and sections, so you may prefer to dip into the book a section at a time, or to look for information on a particular topic by using the contents list and the index. Cross-references in the answers will lead you to more detailed information where this might be helpful, and essential information is repeated whenever it seems to be necessary.

The first part of the book covers the medical management of epilepsy, while the second covers its social management. We have tried to treat these equally, as they are both extremely important and are frequently interlinked. When epilepsy first presents itself, it is usually seen as a medical issue: after all, your first contact is with a doctor. However, it soon becomes apparent that social issues are just as important, and that epilepsy cannot be managed completely successfully without addressing or dealing with both areas.

Not everyone will agree with every answer we have given, but future editions of this book can only be improved by feedback from the people who know most about living with children with epilepsy – in other words, you. If you have any comments about the book, we would be delighted to receive them. It is also very important for us to know of any questions that have not been asked in this book, or of any other topics that you think should have been covered. Please write to us c/o Class Publishing, Barb House, Barb Mews, London W6 7PA.

My child's epilepsy

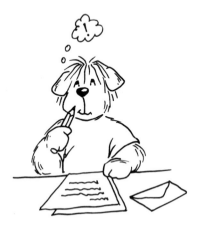

INTRODUCTION

In the main part of this book we explain what epilepsy is, how it is diagnosed and treated, and offer practical suggestions on how to live with it day-to-day. What we do not do there is tell you what it feels like to have or to be a child with epilepsy. That information can only come from families with personal experience, and so we have asked five of them to contribute their own accounts for this preliminary chapter. All the various types of epilepsy they mention are discussed in detail elsewhere in the book.

From Richard's and Joe's mother

We were upset to discover that we had a second son with epilepsy, having coped with it 14 years previously. Our first son was on anti-epileptic drugs between the ages of 5 and 11 but fortunately from then on was free of the epilepsy and the drugs. Our second son started on drugs at about 5 years old, but unfortunately the epilepsy returned after the drugs were withdrawn, so he is now back on the drugs again at age 15.

I must confess I must have appeared a very over-protective parent as I was always watchful over what they participated in and also very persistent over the importance of taking the drugs regularly. However, I always let them do everything they wanted to do (eg swimming and so on) so long as there was always someone with them who was fully aware of the situation, and if I wasn't happy I would go myself to watch.

We found that as they got older their friends were the most reliable support. I always told the teachers but they are so busy that it is difficult to watch every child, and I also felt that some teachers who had never seen an actual attack didn't always take me seriously.

The boys seemed to cope very well, I believe that I was the one most stressed!!! Richard (our older son) says he was never really aware of it at all apart from a headache and what he described as 'weird visual sensations' at the onset of an attack. Joe (our younger son) was getting anxious whilst he was having seizures at 14 and 15 years old but is much happier now that he is on the drugs and stabilised.

I think it is important to try to let them lead life to the full and treat the epilepsy as an irritation to be supervised rather than a disability.

From Joe

By the age of 14 the epileptic absences no longer had any real effect on me as I had grown used to them happening over such a long period of time. Before this my absences would often worry or upset me sometimes and I needed to feel that I was safe from embarrassment. Having good friends and a supportive family were strong comforting factors. However, I would have preferred that people didn't mention it at all and ignored it. This was wrong, though, as only by addressing the problem and getting medication was I able to become virtually clear of the epilepsy.

From Vicky

As I am nearly 16 years old I decided that I wanted to speak for myself instead of letting my parents do it! I was diagnosed with typical childhood onset absence epilepsy when I was 11. At that time I was only young and did not understand what epilepsy was. At first I was quite sick but as time went by I became more able to cope. My Mum, Dad and brother were scared to let me do the things I always loved doing like trampolining, swimming and going out to play with my friends which made me really mad. But when I got used to having epilepsy things got a lot better.

My friends did not treat me any differently but I don't think they really understood how I felt. I wanted friends like me who had epilepsy but I had none – this was hard to explain then and still is now. I then realised I had to think positively. At this stage things got better, more people started understanding which helped me a lot. I did get to meet other boys and girls with epilepsy, and ever since then things have been great. I went away with a group of people with epilepsy, and this made me think differently from the way I'd thought before. I knew for a fact then that I was just the same as everyone else.

My feelings now are totally different – for nearly five years now I have felt happy living with epilepsy. It took a while but I made it and everyone else will too. Right now I have no special feelings about my epilepsy, only that it's there and I have to live with it and take my medication all the time. It hasn't stopped me from doing anything, instead it has given me more confidence and made me more independent. I have been skiing, on school trips to Italy (twice) and Paris (once) and I hope to go to the south of France after my exams next year. When I am older I hope to look after children with epilepsy just as lots of people helped me.

From a lucky mum

Lucky? Yes, we've been really lucky. We've had wonderful help from our consultant, back-up and help from our hospital (luckily we live near) and lucky with our children.

I knew my daughter had epilepsy, so there was no shock with the diagnosis. She has JME – juvenile myoclonic epilepsy. My initial feelings were sympathy, what a shame for my little girl, will she be OK, will she cope? I thought the best advice came from our consultant: 'Do everything, don't let it change your life, let her do it all'. Difficult as it was, and still is, that's just what we did. You put a face on so that the children don't see the feelings behind it, but underneath the worry is awful. One of the worst things is to get the medication correct. You think you've cracked it and then something goes wrong, so you try again. To let go and hope someone else cares as well, that's hard.

My daughter has done everything any other child has done – canoeing, windsurfing, gorge walking, learning to drive, going to discos (even though we worried about the lights). Now we go to concerts where everybody jumps up and down – it's great! I think we worry about most of the things other parents of teenagers worry about, it's just that we have a little extra worry. University and jobs are looming and with those the adult prejudices that we must all cope with, but my daughter is in the front line.

I'm very impressed with how she copes, proud because I don't know whether I would manage as well if it was me, and I'm trying not to think too far ahead about sex, marriage and babies. Just like any other normal parent!

From Jane

My daughter, who has learning difficulties, had had very occasional 'blank spells' as a toddler and a few unexplained falls when at primary school, so it was not a total shock when I received a phone call from the school saying that she had had a fit. She was then 14 years old. Our doctor explained that one attack of this type did not necessarily mean epilepsy, but within a week she had had another fit. Gradually a pattern emerged: a week or so of a cluster of attacks followed by several weeks without a single attack. Despite increased dosages, her anti-epileptic medication did not seem to prevent attacks.

We were aware of the risks of wrapping her in cotton wool, but obviously there were some areas of independence which had to be curtailed. We were also reluctant to leave her with a babysitter so that meant that my husband and I were unable to go out together. We also thought twice about trips out as a family, and during that period we did not take a holiday. The difficulty was the unpredictability of the problem. One day I took my daughter (accompanied by her two younger sisters) to the doctor for a routine check-up and reported to him how well she had been for several weeks; after that we went shopping and my daughter had a drop attack in the supermarket. The staff were very helpful but I was aware that I wanted to drive her home quickly before she had a tonic-clonic seizure (which was what happened after we arrived home).

Several months later, a particularly bad series of attacks resulted in hospitalisation. After this, her medication was changed and since then life has been transformed. My daughter has not had a fit now for 15 months, and during that time we have been away on a family holiday to Florida, involving long flights and coping with a five-hour time-lag and different meal-times. She has also been away on a trip abroad with a group from her school.

No parent likes the idea of long-term medication for their child but we accept it because the alternative is so distressing and potentially dangerous.

From Andrew's mother

We adopted Andrew when he was 6 weeks old. When he was 11 months old I found him having a seizure. I was extremely concerned, never having experienced anything of this sort before. Our GP came immediately, and Andrew was admitted to hospital (he had a high temperature). We spent four days at the hospital until his temperature was back to normal, and in the meantime he cut two teeth. It was explained to us that infants often have febrile convulsions if they have a high temperature. We were told not to worry, he may never have another convulsion and not to think he had epilepsy – very reassuring. Then when he was 13 months old we went on holiday, which involved crossing London. No sooner were we on the Underground than Andrew had a convulsion. We spent four days in a London hospital – again they would not discharge us until his temperature was down. We left with a letter for our GP.

Our GP referred us to a specialist. There was still no mention of epilepsy, but phenobarbitone was prescribed. Andrew took this drug for 18 months, he was just like any normal little boy, albeit a little hyperactive. We had regular appointments with the specialist, who then decided that Andrew did not need the drug any more. He was weaned off the drug over a period of three weeks, and the day after his last dose he had another seizure. He was put back on antiepileptic drugs.

The next four years were horrendous. Andrew fitted more and more, we had weekly appointments with the specialist trying to get the right balance of drugs, we even tried a ketogenic diet. When he was about 4 years old he went into status epilepticus. It later transpired that these fits had caused some brain damage. Our stays at the hospital were terrible, a nightmare, as Andrew became more and more hyperactive, he was into everything and a proper handful. I don't recall anyone ever saying to us that Andrew had epilepsy, I suppose they assumed we knew.

When he was at the age to go to playschool, I took him along to one locally, where they managed him very well for a while, although he did have seizures on a couple of occasions. Our Health Visitor suggested a specialised day nursery might be more suitable, but before I agreed to this I went along to have a chat. I felt it would be right for Andrew; he had a taxi to take him there and collect him. During this time I joined a support group which I found most beneficial. I soon came to realise that I was not the only person in the world who had a child with epilepsy and learning difficulties. We had some wonderful times together and it was through this group that I learned about benefits to which I was entitled (no one else had given me this information).

Just before his fifth birthday, staff from the Education Authority came to assess him to determine what sort of provision he would require and which school would be best suited to his needs. When we had still not heard which school he would be attending, I phoned several times and was told his file had been misplaced and they made arrangements to come and assess him again. When we had still not heard anything several weeks later, I phoned the department several times and was told that they had no record of Andrew at all. I was furious and phoned my solicitor, who was at that time the leader of the County Council. The next day we were given details of the school he was to attend! I requested that we visit the school before his admission, this we did and we were impressed. However, after a few months we were told he could only attend half days, and then the head teacher told us bluntly it was not the correct school for Andrew. We were devastated, and hardly knew where or whom to turn to next.

Our specialist suggested a residential school for Andrew. It was an impressive place, but I couldn't bear the thought of him boarding there, so far from home, seeing him only during school holidays, it almost broke my heart. The specialist agreed, and arranged for Andrew to attend a unit nearer home. We had a look around this school, the staff were very friendly and I felt Andrew would be happy there. He travelled each way by taxi each day – the taxi driver was a super fellow and he always had an escort. For the next six months or so everything was fine.

It was then suggested that Andrew should have an assessment at a specialist unit. He was taken there every Sunday evening and collected and brought home each Friday afternoon. This pattern continued for six long winter months, and the conclusion that they came to was that although Andrew correctly filed in his brain everything he saw or heard, his problem was recalling this information – most probably he would not be able to, or it would be all mixed up – and that he and our whole family would benefit if he went into residential care. Another blow for us. We had been married for 13 years when we adopted Andrew and now he was to go into care. We thought and prayed very hard, and eventually went to have a look at the residential place recommended. It was a lovely place, Andrew was to have his own room and the staff were wonderfully kind. My husband took Andrew there each Sunday and collected him on Friday, and he spent the weekends and all holidays at home – wonderful. We soon all began to benefit from this arrangement.

When Andrew was 11 years old we were asked if we would like for him to live in a house in the community with three other young people and carers to look after them – the answer to a prayer. He settled really well. There were teething troubles at the beginning until the staff became aware of each young person's needs. Andrew and the other three will remain at this house, it is theirs for life. The staff have changed but are all truly wonderful, and Andrew is very happy. There were further problems when he left school at 19 – what was he to do then? He was offered a part-time place at a special centre. He took a while to settle into this new 'job' and to get to know the staff, but things improved and he was offered a full-time place. He now appears very happy both at work and at home. His seizures are well controlled by medication and he no longer sees a consultant. Everything is great, and the staff at his home and his work are more like friends to us.

During the whole of Andrew's life we feel that things have not been explained to us very well (except by our specialist, who was marvellous). Our GP came immediately on request, but at times I felt he was embarrassed about the situation. The Health Visitor was a regular visitor, but not all that helpful. We learnt most about epilepsy by joining the British Epilepsy Association, and our local support group was wonderful. We have felt a lack of support many times, and have encountered numerous difficulties throughout Andrew's life. For most things one has to do battle to obtain satisfaction – bureaucracy works in mysterious ways its wonders to perform!

CHAPTER 1

What is epilepsy?

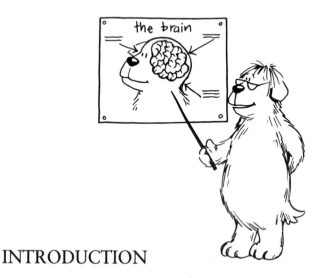

INTRODUCTION

When you first hear people talking about epilepsy you can have the feeling that you are trying to find your way through a maze, with someone speaking in a foreign language as your only guide. Our aim in this chapter is to provide you with a map through the maze, for example by outlining how the brain works, and explaining the many different terms used in epilepsy and how these relate to each other. Obviously every child is different, and so not every term or example we use in this chapter will relate to your child. However, you will come across many of them at one time or another, perhaps when talking to other parents of children with epilepsy (their child's epilepsy may be quite different from your child's).

EPILEPSY AND THE BRAIN

What happens in the brains of people who have epilepsy?

To explain this, we need to start by outlining how the brain works. Many people like to think of the brain and how all its nerve cells work as if it was a very complicated computer full of wires and microchips. Others prefer to think of it as a telephone junction box with wires coming in from thousands and thousands of telephones. However, no one could ever build a computer or telephone junction box that was as good as or that could do as much as the human brain.

The brain is made up of thousands of millions of nerve cells called neurons (we could compare them to the wires in the junction box). Neurons are responsible for controlling all the actions and functions of every part of the body – seeing, hearing, talking, walking and even thinking. As with the computers and junction boxes of our analogy, they work by electricity. Tiny electrical signals are sent along the neurons, between the neurons throughout the brain, and then down into the spinal cord where they can be relayed to any of the other nerves in the body. The links between nerve cells are clearly very important so that they can communicate with each other and pass on the signals.

The actual electrical signals or messages are in the form of chemicals called neurotransmitters ('neuro' means to do with nerve cells and 'transmitters' send or communicate signals or messages). There are many different neurotransmitters within the brain. Some work to cause messages to be sent from one nerve cell to another: these are called excitatory neurotransmitters because they excite or stimulate the neurons. Others work to prevent or stop messages being sent: these are called inhibitory neurotransmitters because they inhibit or hold back the signals. Most of the time there is a very close balance between these different types of neurotransmitters.

As with any complicated machine, the brain can sometimes malfunction or develop faults. In epilepsy the fault usually lies in a loss of balance between the different neurotransmitters. When this happens the electrical signals between the neurons are no longer sent smoothly and in the correct order. Instead they are sent out of order, and this 'out of the correct order' signal then often causes an epileptic seizure. This seizure may take the form of a sudden loss of consciousness, involuntary movements, a change in behaviour or a combination of all of these. (There is more information about seizures in the next two sections of this chapter.)

The drugs used to control epilepsy (called anti-epileptic or anti-convulsant drugs) work by trying to re-establish the correct balance between the different neurotransmitters. The aim is to prevent the 'out of the correct order' electrical signals occurring and so prevent seizures.

Does the same part of the brain go wrong in everyone with epilepsy?

No. The brain is organised into different parts, with each part carrying out different functions (this is discussed further in the answer to the next question). The type of epilepsy and the type of seizure depend on what has gone wrong and in which part of the brain. However, the vast majority of epileptic seizures (probably over 90%) arise from the cerebral hemispheres. Seizures only very rarely start from the cerebellum or the brainstem.

What do the different parts of the brain do?

The human brain has three major parts: the cerebrum, the cerebellum and the brainstem. They are shown in Figure 1.

- **The cerebrum**
  This is by far the largest part of the brain and is divided into halves called cerebral hemispheres. The two hemi-

spheres are joined together by the corpus callosum, which is made up of a large number of nerve fibres. The left hemisphere controls everything that happens down the right-hand side of the body, while the right hemisphere controls what happens down the left-hand side. One hemisphere usually does far more work than the other, although both are clearly important. Whichever does the most work is called the dominant hemisphere. In right-handed people (most of the population), the left hemisphere is dominant; in left-handed people, the right hemisphere is usually the dominant one. The control of speech and language usually lies within the dominant hemisphere.

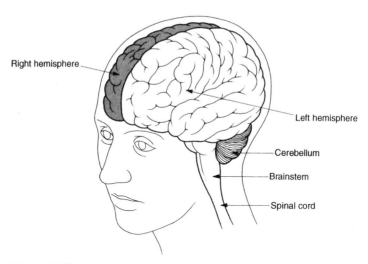

Figure 1: The major parts of the brain.

- **The lobes of the cerebrum**
  Each of the two cerebral hemispheres is divided into four areas: the frontal, parietal, temporal and occipital lobes. They are shown in Figure 2. We still have much to learn about precisely what each lobe does, but we do know

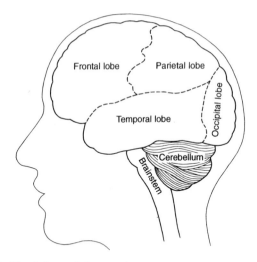

Figure 2: The lobes of the cerebrum.

which lobe is responsible for which of our actions and ways of behaving.

The frontal lobes are involved in the control of our voluntary movements and some aspects of our behaviour and emotions.

The parietal lobes are involved in our perception of touch (feeling) and in control of some of our involuntary movements. They are also involved in skills such as reading, writing and dressing.

The temporal lobes control our speech, language and hearing, our feelings of fear and anger, and our bowel and bladder functions. They are also involved in behaviour.

The occipital lobes are involved in vision and our interpretation of what we see.

- **The cerebellum**
This lies just under the back of the two cerebral hemispheres. It has connections with many other areas of the

brain – including the cerebral hemispheres and the brainstem – and with the spinal cord.

The cerebellum is involved with the control of movements. These may be large or 'gross' movements (such as walking, jumping and running) or small or 'fine' movements (which include drawing, writing, eating and craftwork). The main function of the cerebellum is to enable all these different movements to take place smoothly and fluently by co-ordinating the action of all the different muscles. If the cerebellum is damaged or not working properly, then movements become jerky and clumsy (the medical term for this is ataxia) and a tremor may also develop.

- **The brainstem**
  This very old and very important part of the brain lies right underneath the cerebral hemispheres. It joins all the other parts of the brain to the spinal cord. It was the first part of the brain to evolve – it existed even in prehistoric times and is found in all primates (ie monkeys, apes and humans). Without us being aware of it, it controls breathing and heartbeat, and is involved in the co-ordination of certain activities including swallowing and eye movements. Without the brainstem we would not be able to live – or do anything!

TYPES OF EPILEPSY

Is an epileptic seizure the same thing as a fit?

Yes, and you may also hear seizures referred to as convulsions, attacks or turns. Children often have their own names for seizures ('wobblers' and 'funny do's' seem to be quite popular ones!). They are all used to describe the same thing – a sudden and uncontrolled episode of excessive electrical activity in the brain. The correct, internationally-agreed term for this is seizure, and that is what we have used throughout this book.

Does everyone with epilepsy have the same type of seizure?

No, as there are many different types of seizure. The two main types are called generalised seizures or partial seizures, depending on how much of the brain is involved.

- **Generalised seizures**

  These occur when the abnormal electrical activity that causes a seizure involves both sides of the brain at once, as shown in Figure 3. Generalised seizures can be further divided into six types. It is important to realise that children with epilepsy may have just one type of generalised seizure or they may have many types.

  Absence seizures involve a brief loss of awareness for several (perhaps 5–20) seconds. They usually occur many times a day, every day, and are often accompanied by eyelid fluttering or lip-smacking or chewing movements.

  Myoclonic seizures involve sudden jerky or shock-like contractions of different muscles anywhere in the body, but usually in the arms or legs. Each myoclonic seizure lasts for a fraction of a second, or for one second at most.

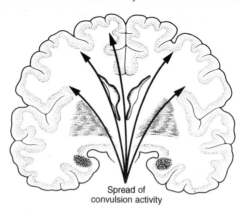

Spread of
convulsion activity

Figure 3: Spread of convulsion activity in a generalised seizure.

Atonic or astatic seizures involve sudden loss of muscle tone (ie sudden relaxation of the muscles) resulting in a fall. They often result in a head injury as the child's head may hit a hard or sharp object such as a desk or table during the fall. An atonic seizure usually lasts for a few seconds, and may be preceded by a very brief myoclonic seizure.

Tonic seizures involve sudden stiffness of the limbs or the whole body, again leading to a fall (often like a tree being felled). The seizure usually ends after 5–10 seconds.

Clonic seizures involve repeated and rhythmic contractions of the muscles, causing jerks or twitches of the limbs or the whole body. They usually last for between 30 seconds and 1–2 minutes, but sometimes last longer.

Tonic-clonic seizures involve a tonic stage followed by a clonic stage, ie sudden stiffness and a fall followed by repeated and rhythmic muscle contractions. Most tonic-clonic seizures last 1–3 minutes; however, some may last for longer, even up to 30 minutes or more (this is then called status epilepticus, and is discussed in more detail in Chapter 4).

- **Partial seizures**
These occur when the abnormal electrical activity starts in one hemisphere, or in one lobe of one hemisphere. Figure 4 shows how starting in the different lobes can determine the sensations felt during a seizure. Partial seizures can be further divided into two types called simple and complex.

'Simple' means that someone's level of consciousness or awareness is not affected during the seizure. Most simple partial seizures involve a change in sensation such as a strange (often unpleasant) smell or taste, or unexplained fear, or a feeling of déjà vu (the 'I've been here before' feeling), or even tingling and numbness in the face

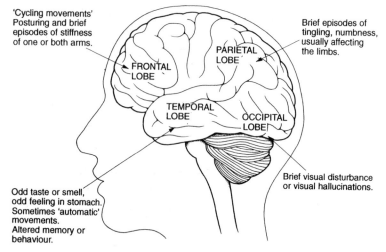

'Cycling movements'
Posturing and brief
episodes of stiffness
of one or both arms.

PARIETAL
LOBE

FRONTAL
LOBE

TEMPORAL
LOBE   OCCIPITAL
              LOBE

Brief episodes of
tingling, numbness,
usually affecting
the limbs.

Brief visual disturbance
or visual hallucinations.

Odd taste or smell,
odd feeling in stomach.
Sometimes 'automatic'
movements.
Altered memory or
behaviour.

Figure 4: Starting in the different lobes determines the sensations felt during a partial seizure.

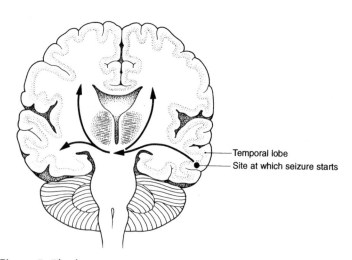

Temporal lobe
Site at which seizure starts

Figure 5: The beginning of a partial seizure in the temporal lobe which may then spread (by way of the arrows) to involve the rest of the brain, resulting in a secondary generalised tonic-clonic seizure.

or an arm. These types of simple partial seizures are called simple partial sensory seizures.

'Complex' means that consciousness or awareness is affected – the person having the seizure may look confused or dazed, or behave or act in a strange way.

If a seizure starts as a partial seizure but then spreads to involve the vast majority of the brain it is called a secondary generalised tonic-clonic seizure (an example of this is shown in Figure 5).

This grouping or classification of the different types of seizure is shown in the diagram in Figure 6.

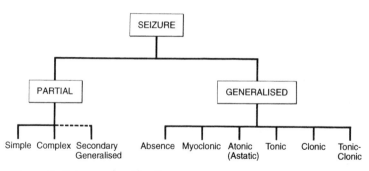

Figure 6: Seizure classification.

So if there are different types of seizure, does that mean there are different types of epilepsy?

Yes, just as there are different types of seizure, so there are different types of epilepsy, also known as epilepsy syndromes. A syndrome is a cluster of signs and symptoms occurring together in a non-fortuitous (ie non-random or non-coincidental) manner. One reason why it is important for doctors to recognise the different types of seizure is that it helps them in turn to recognise different epilepsy syndromes.

Doctors recognise epilepsy syndromes on the basis of four important pieces of information:

- the type of seizure or seizures which the child has (described in the answer to the previous question);
- the age at which the child's seizures started (most epilepsy syndromes are age-related, so some are more likely to occur in infancy, some in middle childhood at 5–10 years of age, some in adolescence, and so on);
- the child's development or learning abilities; and
- what the electroencephalograph (EEG) shows (there is a section on *EEGs* in Chapter 2).

It is only by looking at all of these pieces of information that an epilepsy syndrome can be recognised or identified. However, only about 50%–65% of children will be found to have a clear-cut epilepsy syndrome.

Another way of grouping epilepsy is by how much (if anything) is known about what caused it. Here there are three different groups.

- In idiopathic or primary epilepsy no obvious cause can be found. We suspect that many idiopathic epilepsies may eventually be found to have a genetic basis (discussed in more detail in the section on *Possible causes* later in this chapter).
- In cryptogenic epilepsy a cause is suspected but none can actually be found!
- In symptomatic or secondary epilepsy there is a known cause. For example, the epilepsy may have started after an infection involving the brain (eg meningitis or encephalitis), or after a head injury, or because the brain has never developed properly.

I don't see how all these different classifications fit together. Can you please explain?

Doctors can combine terms from the different classifications to describe a particular type of epilepsy. The description will often include terms describing the cause of the epilepsy, the type of seizure involved and the age when it started. For example, the description 'idiopathic generalised tonic-clonic epilepsy' tells us that the cause is not known (idiopathic), that the seizures affect both sides of the brain (generalised) and that they involve sudden stiffness and a fall followed by repeated rhythmic muscle contractions (tonic-clonic). Similarly the term 'juvenile myoclonic epilepsy' tells us that the epilepsy came on in late childhood or adolescence (the juvenile time of life!) and that the seizures involve jerky muscle contractions (myoclonic).

There are internationally agreed standards for these descriptions, and by following them doctors can ensure that they all know exactly which type of epilepsy is being discussed. Obviously some descriptions will be more common than others, as some types of epilepsy and epilepsy syndromes are more common than others.

Just to make things more complicated, one or two epilepsy syndromes (usually the rarer ones) are known not by these classification descriptions but are instead named after the doctors who first studied them! One example is West syndrome, named after a Dr West who, over 150 years ago, described infantile spasms occurring in his own son. Infantile spasms are a particular type of myoclonic seizure (explained earlier in this section) which usually occur in young children between 3 and 10 months old. The spasms usually occur in clusters, with each cluster consisting of 10–50 spasms or more. The spasms are most often seen when the child wakes up and they may be obvious (affecting the whole body, or the arms and legs) or more subtle (affecting only the head or just the eyelids).

This all strikes me as horribly complicated and I can't see why all these groupings are needed. Why can't we just call it epilepsy and get on with treating it?

You are not alone in finding it complicated – even some

doctors find it a little confusing, particularly those who are not experienced in treating epilepsy. But it is important to try and recognise (ie classify) the specific type of epileptic seizure and the specific epilepsy or epilepsy syndrome, for two main reasons. (When an epilepsy syndrome cannot be identified, then the type of epilepsy is usually classified on the type of seizure.)

The first reason is to give us information on your child's prognosis (ie on the outlook or expected outcome of the child's seizures). You and your doctors need to know whether the seizures will be easily controlled with medication and if there is the possibility that the seizures and the epilepsy may eventually 'go away'. Some types of seizure and some epilepsy syndromes have a better prognosis than others.

The second reason is that knowing which type of epilepsy it is will help guide the doctors in choosing the most appropriate anti-epileptic drug to treat your child. For example, some drugs appear to be more effective in treating partial seizures, whilst others are better at treating generalised seizures.

My GP doesn't use any of the terms you use, he says my son has petit mal. Does this mean my son doesn't actually have epilepsy?

No, it means that your doctor is using an older term for what is now called absence epilepsy. The terms used to describe epilepsy have changed over the years, and although the newer terms are more accurate some people still use the older terms out of habit, or because they sound less technical, or because they are easier to remember. The list that follows gives the modern equivalents for some of the more-commonly used older terms (you will find descriptions of all these types of seizures under their current names earlier in this section).

Old name	Current name
petit mal	absence
jerk	myoclonic
drop	atonic or astatic
stiffening	tonic
repeated jerking	clonic
grand mal	tonic-clonic

My child has been diagnosed as having a benign form of epilepsy. What is this?

'Benign' describes a condition or illness which is not serious and does not usually have harmful consequences. In describing epilepsy it can mean one of two things.

The first is that the seizures are usually controlled very easily with a single anti-epileptic drug – one example of this is an epilepsy syndrome called juvenile myoclonic epilepsy (sometimes referred to as JME from its initials) which may start in late childhood.

The second (and this is the more common reason why the term benign is used) is that the epilepsy usually 'stops' or 'goes away' by itself by late childhood (ie it goes into spontaneous remission). An example of an epilepsy syndrome which does this is benign rolandic epilepsy of childhood (usually abbreviated to BREC).

What is the Lennox-Gastaut syndrome?

This is a specific and rare type of epilepsy syndrome which starts in childhood. The outlook for children with this syndrome is not good (it is the opposite of the benign epilepsies described in the answer to the previous question). These children may need special schooling or, rarely, care in a residential centre for people with severe epilepsy.

It is named after the two eminent experts in epilepsy who first described it. As with any epilepsy syndrome, it has a number of features which help doctors to identify it.

- The age at which the seizures start, which is usually when the child is between 2 and 6 years old. It can occasionally start in children who are 1–2 years old, or in those aged 7 or 8.
- The types of seizures the child has, which are usually of several kinds, including tonic, atonic, tonic-clonic, myoclonic and secondary generalised tonic-clonic seizures (these are all described earlier in this section). The child may also have atypical absence seizures – appearing confused, unresponsive, not talking and perhaps wandering around doing strange things for many minutes (very different from typical absence seizures during which a child simply loses awareness for a number of seconds).
- The EEG shows a characteristic pattern (called slow spike and slow wave activity) which usually occurs over the whole brain and not just one part of it (EEGs are discussed in more detail in Chapter 2).

There are many different causes of Lennox-Gastaut syndrome, for example an abnormal development of the brain before birth or following on from meningitis as a baby, or brain damage occurring around the time of birth. Some children with this syndrome will have had another rare type of epilepsy called infantile spasms or West syndrome in their first year of life and will then go on to have the Lennox-Gastaut syndrome before their second or third birthday. However, a definite cause will only be found in about 50%–60% of the children with the syndrome.

Unfortunately this is a severe form of epilepsy. The seizures are very difficult to control and very few children ever have all the different seizure types fully controlled for more than a few weeks or months at a time. Because of this, most of the anti-epileptic drugs are tried, often in combination with each other. The ketogenic diet (described in more detail in the section on *Diet* in Chapter 3) is also sometimes tried but is not always successful. If the child has very frequent atonic or tonic-clonic seizures (often occurring many times a day) then a surgical procedure called a corpus callosotomy may occasionally be considered. This involves division of the corpus callosum, the part of the brain which joins together the two cerebral hemispheres, and it may in some children result in stopping these types of seizures or at least reducing their frequency.

The child's learning and behaviour will also be affected. Almost 90% of children who have Lennox-Gastaut syndrome will already have had development problems or learning difficulties when the seizures start. After one, two or three years of having seizures, all children with the syndrome have learning and behaviour difficulties – often severe. This usually happens even if the child's seizures are quite well-controlled.

MORE ABOUT SEIZURES

Can you have seizures without having epilepsy?

Yes, and many people will have at least one seizure during their lives. Doctors will only diagnose epilepsy if seizures have been unprovoked and have occurred two or three times. The diagnosis of epilepsy is discussed in Chapter 2.

My son twitches a lot when he is concentrating. Could he have epilepsy?

Episodes of unusual involuntary movements during which consciousness (awareness) is not affected are not always seizures. Seizures are usually spontaneous and self-limiting. If your son's involuntary movements only happen at certain times (eg when he is concentrating or when he is anxious) and if his consciousness is unaffected, then it is more likely that he has a 'tic' or a habit spasm or a mannerism than that he has epilepsy. However, it is important to make the correct diagnosis so we would suggest that you discuss it with your GP if you think that it may be more than a simple tic.

The most common tics which affect children include blinking, shoulder-shrugging, head-shaking and foot-stamping. They appear to be more common in boys than in girls, and there is no medical treatment for them. It is important not to make too much fuss about these movements but you may need to reassure your son that he will grow out of them (if he has even noticed them himself). If tics or habit spasms are frequent and are causing a child distress (eg teasing or bullying at school, or loss of sleep) then it may be necessary to get professional help, perhaps from a child psychologist or psychiatrist.

What about turning the head to one side? Is that a type of seizure or is it simply one of these tics you've described?

It could perhaps be a tic, but it could also be a type of seizure called an adversive seizure. As we said in the answer to the previous question, distinguishing between tics and seizures is important, so if you are in any doubt we would suggest you talk to your doctor.

In an adversive seizure the eyes or head (or both) turn slowly to one side. The body may then begin to turn in the same direction, almost as if walking in a circle. An adversive seizure is usually a complex partial seizure, and it may be followed by a secondary generalised tonic-clonic seizure. Much less commonly an adversive seizure is simply the BEGINNING of a generalised tonic-clonic seizure. (You will find more information on all these types of seizure elsewhere in this section and in the previous section on *Types of epilepsy*.)

Our daughter doesn't twitch or shake or fall down or do any of the other things that we thought were involved in epilepsy. All she does is stare into space sometimes, so why do the doctors want to do tests to see if she has epilepsy?

Many children, especially young children, have episodes of staring into space or day-dreaming and in the majority of cases this is all it is. However, there are occasions when these episodes give rise for concern, perhaps when a teacher reports a tailing-off in the quality of school work by a child who was doing well previously. In this situation, absence seizures (which involve a brief loss of consciousness for some 5–20 seconds) must be considered. We don't know what led you to talk to the doctors about your daughter's episodes of staring into space, but we agree with them that it is worth doing some tests to find out whether or not she has epilepsy. EEGs are the crucial investigative test for this particular form of epilepsy, and there is a section about them in Chapter 2.

Can children get warnings of seizures?

Yes, children whose epilepsy starts from any of the lobes of the brain (but particularly the temporal lobe) often experience a warning that a seizure is about to happen (the lobes of the brain are shown in Figure 2 earlier in this chapter). This warning usually involves a strange sensation, feeling, smell or taste and is known as an 'aura'. An aura is actually a simple partial sensory seizure (explained in the previous section on *Types of epilepsy*). The most common warning sensations are:

- pins and needles (paraesthesia) in one or more limbs, which may spread up the limb, eg from the toes to the hip, or from the fingers to the shoulder and face;
- epigastric sensations (unpleasant feelings or sensations in the stomach);
- gustatory-olfactory sensations (strange tastes or smells);
- fear or panic;
- a feeling of déjà vu (the 'I've been here before' feeling);
- visual or auditory hallucinations (seeing or hearing strange things).

Is there anything that can trigger a seizure?

Failing to take anti-epileptic drugs regularly, becoming

overtired, hyperventilation (overbreathing, ie breathing too fast or too deeply) and having a high temperature or fever are all examples of situations where a seizure may be more likely to happen. In that sense we could say that these examples could be considered 'triggers' for epilepsy.

However, there is also a rare group of epilepsies called reflex epilepsies in which a seizure can occur in response to a specific trigger or stimulus. The best-known of these (because it has received so much media publicity in the last few years) is photosensitivity, and this is discussed in the answer to the next question. Very few children have reflex epilepsy: even if they do, they rarely encounter any of the triggering factors.

I remember seeing a lot of reports on the television about the flashing patterns in computer games bringing on epilepsy. My son has seizures, so will these affect him?

Only if he is photosensitive. Photosensitivity means being sensitive or susceptible to flashing or flickering lights, but only when the flashes or flickers occur at a certain frequency. It may occur in isolation but is far more commonly seen in children (and adults) who have epilepsy – usually idiopathic (also called primary) generalised epilepsy (explained in the previous section in this chapter). However, only about 5% of children with epilepsy are photosensitive. Photosensitivity usually develops at between 6 and 18 years of age, with a peak at 12–16 years old, and it tends to affect girls more often than boys. Most children who are photosensitive will grow out of it by their early or mid-twenties.

Seizures can be triggered in children with photosensitive epilepsy by:

- flashing lights (often with 12–20 flashes per second);
- strobe lighting (often found in discos or amusement arcades);
- sunlight shining through a row of trees, railings or

buildings as the child passes by in a car or bus or, occasionally, if the child is running fast past them;
• strongly striped or geometric patterns.

It is important to realise that flashing lights, television sets and computer games do NOT make a child photosensitive or cause epilepsy. They are only able to trigger or provoke a seizure in a child who is already susceptible, or who already has epilepsy. In fact, only about 4%–5% of ALL people with epilepsy are photosensitive, and because of this only a small number of children with epilepsy may be affected by the flashing patterns on computers.

Doctors can find out whether or not your son is photosensitive by performing an EEG, and this test is described in the section on *EEGs* in Chapter 2. If he is, then there are sections on practical ways of handling *Discos*, *Television* and *Computers and computer games* in Chapter 9.

My baby daughter has epilepsy and she is due to have her vaccinations soon. I've heard that vaccinations can make seizures worse, so should we say that we don't want her to have them?

No, you shouldn't, as the great majority of children who have epilepsy can be vaccinated (immunised). Having epilepsy is not a reason for not having vaccinations and this is equally true for anyone in the family who has epilepsy (mother, father, brother, sister, uncle, aunt, grandmother or grandfather or cousin – even the family pet!).

All the usual vaccinations are considered to be safe for children with epilepsy, including polio, tetanus, diphtheria, whooping cough (also called pertussis), MMR (which stands for measles, mumps and rubella – rubella is another name for German measles) and BCG (the vaccine for tuberculosis). There are only two definite reasons for a child (with or without epilepsy) not to be vaccinated. The first is if the child has had a bad (adverse) reaction to a previous dose of the same vaccine: it is very rare for this to happen. The second is if the child is unwell at the time when the vaccination is due to be given – and this is only a reason for delaying the vaccination, not for not having it at all.

Giving the vaccine (whichever one it is) will be straightforward and not cause a problem for over 99% of children with epilepsy. However, for a few children, particularly those with severe epilepsy, the number of seizures may increase for a time just after the vaccination. This is because there may be a rise in temperature and a mild illness after the vaccine has been given, something which is particularly likely to happen about 8–10 days after a measles or MMR vaccination. This is still not a reason for not having the vaccination, as seizures can also increase during any illness or infection, including the common cold, influenza and gastroenteritis. More unusually, seizures may actually become less during one of these infections!

We keep being told that children lead more stressful lives these days, that they have to grow up so quickly and so on. How does this affect children with epilepsy like my son – will it make him have more seizures?

Stress in itself rarely provokes a seizure. However, if your son is in a stressful situation (eg worrying about exams or family problems) then this may well have an adverse effect on his sleeping pattern and general health, which in turn may lower his seizure threshold and make a seizure more likely to happen.

We all need to develop ways of handling stress, whether or not we have epilepsy – it is a natural part of life and it is impossible for any of us to avoid it completely. Your worry that stress will provoke your son's seizures is very natural, but it will not actually do either of you very much good. It would be better to talk to him about his worries and decide between you how he can best cope with them. You can also help by encouraging him to look after his general health, for example by making sure that he eats a healthy diet and takes regular exercise.

Lyndsay's epilepsy is much worse around her periods. Is there a reason for this?

Some women and girls complain that their seizures are worse at the start of or just before their periods. Seizures which are caused or made worse by menstruation (periods) are called catamenial seizures (from the Greek word 'katamenios' which means monthly). Lyndsay's specialist may be able to adjust her anti-epileptic drugs to allow for her catamenial seizures.

It is possible that cyclical changes in seizure frequency may well be related to specific times in the monthly menstrual cycle. One suggested cause is the rapid fall in levels of progesterone (one of the female sex hormones) which naturally occurs at or immediately before a period. It is also thought that the fluid retention which some women and girls have then may also play a part in making seizures worse, and some doctors will prescribe diuretics (drugs which increases the flow of urine, often known as water tablets) during this part of the cycle.

Our teenage son went to a party the other night and got drunk for the first time in his life. He then had a seizure. Does alcohol effect epilepsy and, if so, will he have to stop drinking it completely?

Alcohol is in fact a drug and therefore anyone who drinks it may be affected by it. It can make anti-epileptic medication less effective and may actually cause seizures if too much is drunk at one time, although an occasional drink is unlikely to be harmful.

Because drinking alcohol is seen as a symbol of sociability, it is important for young people to find their own levels and to avoid drinking too much. Your son will probably not have to stop drinking alcohol completely, but he will need to get the balance right – this will not only involve thinking about the amount that he drinks, but also his sleeping (particularly important) and eating patterns (both easily disrupted by too much alcohol).

As medical research suggests that drinking more than two units of alcohol increases the risk of seizures in people with epilepsy, a sensible daily limit would appear to be about one or at most two units. A unit of alcohol is equivalent to one glass of wine OR half a pint of average strength beer or lager OR one single measure of spirits. Saving up a daily alcohol 'allowance' for a weekend binge (ie drinking 7–14 units over the weekend) would be a mistake and would almost certainly increase the risk of your son having a seizure.

Can children have epilepsy in their sleep?

Yes, children can have seizures during sleep. Some children only ever have seizures when they are asleep at night and never during the day when they are awake. Some types of epilepsy are commonly associated with seizures that occur during sleep or just after waking: examples include benign myoclonic epilepsy of infancy; benign rolandic epilepsy of childhood (BREC); juvenile myoclonic epilepsy (JME); and complex partial seizures (particularly if they arise from the frontal lobes).

Because most people sleep at night, these seizures are described as nocturnal seizures (from the Latin word 'nocturnus' meaning 'during the night'), although they can occur whenever someone is asleep. We do not yet know the reason for them, but we do know that when the brain is relatively inactive (as during some parts of sleep), then it is more likely that a seizure will occur. This is why EEG tests are sometimes done during sleep or after a period of sleep deprivation – it increases the chance of abnormal electrical signals showing up (there is a section on *EEGs* in Chapter 2).

Why does my daughter wet herself when she has a seizure?

It is difficult to give you a precise reason without knowing what type of seizure your daughter has, but we can give you a general answer. Children can wet themselves during two types of seizure. The first and more common of these is a generalised tonic-clonic seizure, because during this type of seizure there can be a sudden and often disordered contraction of the abdominal and bladder muscles. If these contractions are very disordered there can even be some faecal incontinence, ie when children can dirty or soil themselves.

The other type of seizure in which urinary incontinence can occur (ie when children wet themselves) is a complex partial seizure, although this is uncommon. In this type of seizure children are not fully aware of where they are or what they are doing, and so they may try and urinate (pass water) inappropriately, ie in the wrong place and at the wrong time.

Both the types of seizure mentioned in this answer are discussed in more detail elsewhere in this section and in the previous section on *Types of epilepsy*.

I was talking to another mother in the hospital waiting room, and her son's seizures sounded different from my daughter's. But we'd both been told that our children have complex partial seizures, so why the differences?

Our explanation has to be very general, because we don't know enough about either child to be more specific. You have been told that your daughter has complex partial seizures – 'complex' meaning that she has some loss of or alteration in her consciousness (awareness) during a seizure, and 'partial' meaning that her seizures start in only one part of her brain (these terms are explained in more detail in the section on *Types of epilepsy* earlier in this chapter). The differences that you and the other mother have noticed suggest that although your children both have complex partial seizures, these seizures may be starting in different places in the brain. Exactly where in the brain a seizure starts will determine what happens during it.

Complex partial seizures can occasionally start in one or other of the frontal lobes (the different lobes are shown in Figure 2 in the section on *Epilepsy and the brain* earlier in this chapter). However, they USUALLY start in the temporal lobes, which is why you may sometimes hear the description 'temporal lobe epilepsy'. The temporal lobes control emotion, memory, speech and language (among other things): exactly what happens during a complex partial seizure will depend upon which part of the temporal lobe is involved. The seizures may be associated with unexpected movements, strange feelings, fluctuating emotions or altered behaviour. As well as this, complex partial seizures may spread to involve the whole brain, when they are known as secondary generalised tonic-clonic seizures and have different effects again.

My grandson is the only child I know with epilepsy. When he has a seizure he goes unconscious, falls down and then shakes all over. Is this typical – do all children with epilepsy do this?

As you can see from other answers in this chapter, there are many different types of seizure, so the answer to the second part of your question is no, not all children have the type of seizure you describe.

Coming back to the first part of your question, your grandson's seizures are typical of a particular type of epilepsy called generalised tonic-clonic seizures. During this type of seizure the child's body will stiffen, there may be a cry (this is not pain) or grunt followed by a fall, and then the convulsion begins. Your grandson may go blue (cyanosed) because of lack of oxygen, he may drool or froth at the mouth (also called salivation), he may wet himself, and there will be rhythmic jerking movements of all his limbs (the shaking you describe).

This type of seizure usually lasts between one and three minutes and usually stops by itself. Occasionally, in very severe cases, drugs such as diazepam (brand names for this drug include Valium, Diazemuls and Stesolid) may have to be given to stop the seizure. There is more information about this treatment in the sections on *Anti-epileptic drugs* in Chapter 3 and on *First aid* in Chapter 4.

Why does he turn blue during a seizure?

Not all children turn blue during a generalised tonic-clonic seizure, but it can occasionally happen. When it occurs, it is usually most noticeable around the lips and mouth (it is then called perioral cyanosis).

The blueness is due to the fact that during the seizure his breathing becomes irregular and because of this not enough oxygen fills his lungs. When this happens the blood going to all his tissues and organs (including the skin, which is an organ) is not quite as pink as it usually is, and therefore the skin can turn a little blue. Usually it only takes two or three minutes for breathing to become more regular, and then the oxygen within the lungs and within the blood rapidly becomes normal and the skin quickly turns pink again.

Do seizures change as children grow up?

This can often happen, particularly if the seizures started in the first couple of years of life. In some children the epilepsy 'goes away' as they grow up (eg benign rolandic epilepsy of childhood), but in others it persists into adolescence and adult life (eg juvenile myoclonic epilepsy). The type and frequency of seizures may change in the teenage years because of a number of factors, including:

- the natural history of the particular epilepsy or epilepsy syndrome (ie what usually happens in that type of epilepsy);
- the influence of age and hormones, eg puberty, the menarche (when menstrual periods start);

- the effects of a typically erratic teenage lifestyle (a very busy social life, including the use of alcohol and a disturbed sleep pattern);
- forgetting or refusing to take anti-epileptic drugs regularly;
- the development of photosensitivity as the child gets older (photosensitivity was discussed earlier in this section).

Are there any risks of long-term damage to health from having seizures?

This is a difficult question to answer as so many factors have to be taken into consideration, including the type of epilepsy the child has, what is known about its cause, and whether the child has any other medical problems as well as epilepsy. At one end of the scale there are children who have seizures only occasionally, and of a type which usually 'goes away' as they grow up: for them, we can say that there are few or no risks of any long-term health damage. At the other end of the scale are children with severe epilepsy and other major problems, and for them we can only say that the risks are much greater. In general, the effects of epilepsy on a child's long-term health will be less favourable in the following circumstances:

- if the epilepsy began when the child was under 2 years old;
- if the cause of the epilepsy is known, eg lack of oxygen to a baby's brain at birth, or a complication of meningitis or encephalitis, or because the brain never developed properly before birth;
- if the child has associated neurological abnormalities or disorders (ie other problems affecting the brain or nervous system), learning difficulties or developmental delay (ie the child's physical, mental, emotional and social skills are not developing as they should);
- if the type of seizure includes myoclonic, tonic or atonic

seizures (these types of seizure are described in the section on *Types of epilepsy* earlier in this chapter);

- if initial seizure control was difficult;
- if more than one anti-epileptic drug is needed to control the seizures;
- if the child has episodes of convulsive status epilepticus (see Chapter 4 for more information about status epilepticus).

POSSIBLE CAUSES

Do we know what causes epilepsy?

In most cases, no. In almost 75% of all children diagnosed as having epilepsy, no specific cause for it will be found. This is why so many types of epilepsy are described as being 'idiopathic', which simply means that the cause is not known. (Idiopathic comes from two Greek words, 'idios' meaning own and 'pathos' meaning suffering). It seems likely that some of these idiopathic forms of epilepsy may have a genetic cause, and this is discussed in the answer to the next question.

In a minority of children we do know the reason why they have developed epilepsy. Epilepsy can be due to virtually anything which affects the brain, and seizures may also occur in association with many other disorders which do not affect the brain directly. For example, epilepsy may start after an infection involving the brain (eg meningitis or encephalitis), or after a head injury, or because the brain has never developed properly, or because of cerebral hypoxia (lack of oxygen to the baby's brain) at birth. When a cause is known, the epilepsy is described as being 'symptomatic' or 'secondary'.

Can you inherit epilepsy?

A lot of research is going on at the moment into the links between different medical conditions (not just epilepsy) and our genetic makeup (the characteristics we inherit from our parents). More and more conditions are turning out to have a genetic cause, and epilepsy is probably no different. There are many different types of epilepsy (as we explained in the previous section in this chapter), and some of these types of epilepsy may have a genetic basis.

Genes are the parts of a human cell which determine which characteristics you inherit from your parents. In other words, the cells in your body contain sets of instructions (genes) which control the ways in which the cells grow and behave. Things can go wrong with these sets of instructions (they are then called abnormal genes), and it may be that one or more abnormal genes are responsible for causing epilepsy. If a child happens to inherit one or more of these abnormal genes from their parents, then the child may develop epilepsy. The particular genes a child gets from each parent are a matter of chance, and this applies just as much to abnormal genes as to the ones which determine the colour of our eyes or the size of our feet.

It is also important to realise that one or both parents may simply be carrying one of the abnormal genes without necessarily having epilepsy themselves. In this situation, epilepsy may still develop in their child or children.

We do know that inheritance plays a part in one particular type of epilepsy called primary generalised epilepsy. If someone in the family (a parent or a brother or sister) has this type of epilepsy, then the chances of another child in the family having a similar type of epilepsy are increased by about 10 times. If there is no family history of this type of epilepsy, then a child has at most a 0.5%–1% chance of developing it (ie approximately one child in every 100–200 children) but if someone in the close family already has it, then the chances increase to 5%–10% (ie approximately one child in every 10–20 children). Other types of epilepsy and other epilepsy syndromes carry different, and often much lower risks.

Can other conditions which affect the brain cause epilepsy?

Epilepsy is far more common in children (and adults) who have other conditions which affect the brain. These conditions include cerebral palsy (25%–30% of children with cerebral palsy have epilepsy), learning difficulties (up to 50% of children with severe learning difficulties have epilepsy), and behaviour problems including autism (about 30% of autistic children have epilepsy). All of these conditions have different causes, but the common link between them is a brain abnormality, ie something has gone wrong in the brain or the brain has been damaged in some way. It is the brain abnormality, whatever its cause, which is responsible for causing all these problems, including any epilepsy. However, none of these conditions actually CAUSES epilepsy, and neither does epilepsy cause cerebral palsy, learning difficulties, behaviour problems and so on.

Unfortunately, the epilepsy which occurs in association with any of these other medical conditions is likely to be more severe and more difficult to control with anti-epileptic drugs. Conditions which are usually linked to difficult epilepsy include cerebral palsy, tuberous sclerosis and severe learning difficulties. Infections which affect the brain (eg meningitis or encephalitis) may also lead to difficult epilepsy.

Epilepsy may also be caused by a head injury, although this is rare. It usually follows only a bad or serious head injury which led to a long period of unconsciousness or loss of memory; or one in which the skull was fractured and the edge of the broken skull bone was forced downwards into the brain; or one which caused a blood clot to develop in the brain.

In children, brain tumours only very rarely cause epilepsy. Out of every 100 children with epilepsy, only one or two will be found to have a brain tumour. In adults, the figure is more likely to be 20 or 30.

Every so often there are newspaper reports about children becoming brain damaged after having whooping cough vaccine. Does the vaccine cause epilepsy?

Nearly all the medical evidence suggests that the answer to your question is a clear 'no'. In fact, there is a much greater risk of brain damage and epilepsy occurring in a young child (one less than 2 or 3 years old) who has NOT been vaccinated against whooping cough (also called pertussis) than of a child of a similar age suffering brain damage because of the vaccine.

A very few children have appeared to develop epilepsy after a vaccination. In these children, the seizures have usually started suddenly, within 12–24 hours of them being vaccinated. We do not know the reason for this, but one suggestion is that there may have been a fault in the way that a particular batch or supply of the vaccine was manufactured. The chances of such a thing happening are extremely rare (the reason it is reported in the newspapers is because it is so rare and therefore considered newsworthy) and it cannot be considered a reason for a child not to be vaccinated. Vaccination has been so effective in controlling childhood illnesses that we have almost forgotten how dangerous some of these infections can be.

Some children who have never had a seizure in their lives may have a febrile (feverish) fit or convulsion after a vaccination. Once again this is a very rare occurrence, but if it does happen it is most likely to take place 8–10 days after a measles or MMR (measles, mumps, rubella) vaccination. It is important to realise that this febrile convulsion is NOT epilepsy and that the child will usually never have another seizure.

FACTS AND FIGURES

How many children have epilepsy?

In this country, approximately 350,000–400,000 people of

all ages currently have epilepsy, and of these some 90,000–
100,000 are children aged anywhere from a few months old
to 16 years old. This means that epilepsy affects some 5–8
children in any thousand. As the proportion of a population
with a particular medical condition at any one time is
referred to as the 'prevalence', we could say that the
prevalence of epilepsy among children in this country is
0.5%–0.8%.

The 'incidence' of a condition is the number of people
developing it for the first time during each year (ie the
number of new cases within a year). In children the incidence of epilepsy varies, depending upon the age of the
child. It is highest in the first year of life: in any one year
approximately 140 children in every 100,000 who are
under a year old will be diagnosed with epilepsy. This figure
falls to 70 children in every 100,000 between the ages of 5
and 10, and to 40 children in every 100,000 between the
ages of 10 and 20.

How many of these children with epilepsy go on to be adults with epilepsy?

Epilepsy is most likely to develop in the first 16 years of life,
so it is not surprising to find that almost one half (50%) of
all adults with epilepsy first had it in childhood. However, it
is also important to realise that of ALL the children
developing epilepsy under the age of 16 years, in one third
(about 33%) it will stop (this is called spontaneous remission) and seizures will never happen again in adult life.

Is there more epilepsy around these days? If so, is there anything we can do to prevent it?

Epilepsy does not appear to be on the increase. A small
proportion of epilepsy is preventable, for example by taking
sensible safety measures to protect children from severe
head injuries or by treating quickly any infections which
may affect the brain (eg meningitis or encephalitis). How-

ever, as we do not know the cause of most epilepsy (although we suspect it may have a genetic basis – see the previous section on *Possible causes* for more about this), it is largely unpreventable.

Is epilepsy more common in girls than in boys, or vice versa?

When you look at all types of epilepsy at all ages, there is no difference between males and females in terms of the incidence or prevalence of epilepsy (figures for incidence and prevalence are given in an earlier answer in this section). However, there are certain types of epilepsy which are more common in females than in males, for example absence epilepsy. Photosensitivity is also more common in females.

Is it true that epilepsy is linked to high intelligence?

No. It is important to realise that epilepsy can occur in children who have below average, average or above average intelligence. However, children who have brain damage or children in whom the brain has never developed properly and who have learning difficulties or cerebral palsy (or both) are much more likely to have a severe form of epilepsy and also to have seizures which may persist for most of their lives.

CHAPTER 2

Diagnosing epilepsy

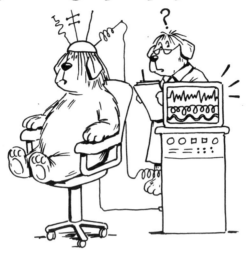

INTRODUCTION

It is obviously crucial to establish a correct diagnosis of epilepsy, as without this it would be impossible for your child's doctor to plan which investigations needed to be done, decide which treatment will be most suitable or predict what might happen in the future. The diagnosis of epilepsy may be either easy or difficult to make. There is no one test which will absolutely confirm or deny epilepsy, so doctors have to take many factors into account. This can mean that the process of diagnosis can sometimes seem long and frustrating. Understanding what is going on can help to make the process feel less tedious, and we hope that the explanations in this chapter will help with this.

HOW DO THEY KNOW IT'S EPILEPSY?

What tests are needed to diagnose epilepsy?

The diagnosis of epilepsy is always a clinical diagnosis, ie it is mainly based on what the doctor is told and on the information you and your child provide (you will be asked a great many questions!). EEGs can provide useful additional information, particularly about the type of epilepsy or epilepsy syndrome, and a few children may need brain scans. There are separate sections on *EEGs* and *Scans* later in this chapter; in this section we concentrate on the information the doctors need to make a clinical diagnosis of epilepsy.

Making a correct clinical diagnosis of epilepsy can take some time, and it is very unlikely that any harm will come to your child by waiting. It is very important that the diagnosis is correct, as a wrong diagnosis can lead to future problems. If your child has only had one unprovoked epileptic seizure, then most doctors agree that no further investigation is necessary. Should a second or third seizure occur, then your GP will probably refer you to a specialist at your local hospital. Most children will be seen at the hospital within 4–6 weeks, and some are seen earlier than this.

I didn't actually see my son have a seizure, it was his older sister who told me what had happened. I will be the person taking him to the doctor, but should my daughter come along as well?

Yes, she should. Before a diagnosis can be made, a doctor needs to be given a very clear, detailed and accurate account of precisely what happened to a child during a seizure. It is therefore essential that the person who has actually seen the child having the seizure (the eyewitness) should go along to give the doctor this very important information. In your son's case, the eyewitness is your daughter.

Your doctor will have to ask many questions about what actually happened before, during and after your son's seizure. The sequence of events should be described as accurately as possible. If this information (called the history) is unclear or incomplete, then a diagnosis of epilepsy must not be made and the doctor must wait for more information. The most common reason for a mistaken or wrong diagnosis of epilepsy is that someone has failed to take a detailed and accurate history of what happened to a child during a seizure and has then jumped to the wrong conclusion. Usually this is because no one can remember what happened just before the seizure began.

Your daughter should not worry if she is unable to remember every detail of what happened to your son (she would be an exceptional person if she could!). She should simply do her best to answer your doctor's questions as fully as possible.

All I can remember about my daughter's first seizure is being in a complete state of panic, I was so frightened. I managed to call the doctor, but I simply wasn't able to describe properly what had happened. Did I do the right thing?

Yes, you did. It is not surprising that in the circumstances you were unable to remember every detail of what happened to your daughter, and the way you felt was not unusual. A number of research studies have clearly shown that when parents see their child's first tonic-clonic seizure they actually think that the child is going to die, and they feel utterly helpless. This common response indicates the degree of anxiety felt by parents when a child has a seizure. It is important to realise that it is rare for anyone to die during a seizure.

When a child has a seizure for the first time, the GP should be asked to see the child, preferably as soon as possible. In the vast majority of children the seizure will have stopped by the time that the doctor gets there. If for some reason the GP is not available then it is entirely reasonable to call an ambulance and have the child taken to the

Accident and Emergency (casualty) department of the nearest hospital. If a seizure lasts for more than 10–15 minutes then this is an emergency and an ambulance must be called immediately (there is more about emergencies in Chapter 4).

How does anyone ever remember enough details about a seizure to be able to describe it to a doctor?

It is very common for eyewitnesses (whether they be parents, brothers, sisters, friends or school teachers) not to be able to remember exactly what happened when a child had a seizure. Eyewitnesses seeing a seizure for the first time may be understandably frightened and may actually think that the child is going to die (something which only rarely happens), and because of this they cannot remember the exact sequence of events. And by the time the child has been taken to see a specialist at a hospital, it may have been some days or even weeks since the seizure and the eyewitnesses may have forgotten what actually happened. Doctors are well used to this happening, and will usually ask questions to jog the eyewitnesses' memories and help them remember as many details as possible.

If you can overcome your initial panic, then when your child has another seizure it would be useful for you to write down as soon as you can all the details of what happened in the exact order in which they occurred. Another very useful way of providing an accurate description of a seizure is to actually film or record one with a camcorder (if you have one). Your child's specialist would find such a video extremely useful, not only to help in making a correct diagnosis of epilepsy but also in establishing the specific type of seizure and epilepsy. Miming or acting out how your child moved or behaved during a seizure can also help, as it is often easier to show a doctor what happened than to try and describe it in words. The doctor may even do the miming for you!

Our family doctor is very good at discussing things with us and she always explains exactly what is going on. When we told her about our son's first seizure, she said she was not sure whether or not it was epilepsy, although it might be, so she is referring us to a specialist at the hospital. Why doesn't she know for sure – is it very difficult for doctors to diagnose epilepsy?

Yes, it can be. The first problem is that there are a number of other conditions which can produce episodes or attacks which may resemble or look like an epileptic seizure (they are discussed in the answer to the next question). It is obviously very important for a doctor to know that these conditions exist and what may happen to the child if he has one. However, as family doctors have to know a lot about many different conditions, it is not surprising that many GPs do not know about these specific ones in detail, in particular the similarities and differences between the attacks caused by them and the attacks caused by epilepsy.

Another reason why it may be difficult to make a precise diagnosis is that there are many different types of epileptic seizure, and many different types of epilepsy and epilepsy syndromes. Some seizures are very obvious and are easily recognised, for example a generalised tonic-clonic seizure or an atonic seizure (all the different types of seizure mentioned here are discussed in more detail in Chapter 1). Other seizures may be more subtle and therefore more difficult to recognise, for example a brief absence seizure (where a child may just appear to stare into space for some seconds), a brief myoclonic seizure (which may be simply a sudden or momentary jerk of the head or body) or a complex partial seizure (which may just show itself by the child appearing a little confused and behaving rather strangely).

As we have explained in the earlier answers in this section, the information that is most needed in making a diagnosis of epilepsy is a precise description of what happened during a seizure, and eyewitnesses cannot always remember the exact details. When you take all these factors into account, it is not surprising that your GP was a little unsure about making a firm diagnosis. She therefore did the sensible thing and referred you for a second opinion (ALL children with suspected epilepsy should be seen by a specialist).

The specialist that you and your son see may be a paediatrician (a doctor who specialises in treating children), a neurologist (one who specialises in the brain and nervous system) or a paediatric neurologist (a neurologist who concentrates on, and works only with children): it will depend on the way the hospital is organised. Whatever the label, the specialist will have a wider understanding and knowledge of the different sorts of epilepsy than your GP, and should be able to decide whether your son has epilepsy or some other non-epileptic condition. Clearly, this sounds far quicker and easier than it will be in real life! The diagnosis of epilepsy is never a snap judgement. Instead, as you would expect, the specialist will need to ask a lot of questions and perhaps carry out some tests before making a definite diagnosis.

Which other conditions affecting children can be mistaken for epilepsy?

Of the conditions listed below, reflex anoxic seizures and breath-holding attacks are the ones most commonly mistaken for epilepsy in young children. Fainting, migraine, hyperventilation and pseudoseizures (also called pseudo-epileptic seizures or non-epileptic attacks) are the most common causes of misdiagnosis in older children.

- **Jitteriness in a newborn baby**

- **Benign neonatal (newborn) sleep myoclonus**
  This can occur in babies and infants under 7 or 8 months old – they will have occasional jerks of the arms, legs or body ONLY when they are asleep. Similar jerks occur in

older children and adults as they are falling asleep: these are called hypnagogic or hypnic jerks and are NOT myoclonic epileptic seizures.

- **Blue breath-holding attacks**
  Breath-holding attacks are common in toddlers aged between 15 months and 3 years. If they are told off or frustrated by not being able to do something they will cry, then usually deliberately hold their breath and become cyanosed or blue. They may lose consciousness very briefly and then go limp. The whole episode lasts 1–2 minutes and children usually recover very quickly.

- **Reflex anoxic seizures**
  Also called pallid syncopal attacks, these are common in young children, often aged between 15 months and 4 or 5 years, although they may also occur in older children. Following a sudden fright or a sudden pain (such as trapping a finger in a door or banging the back of the head), the child will suddenly cry, become very pale, and may stiffen and then go limp. There may be one or two brief jerks of the arms or legs. After a few seconds or a minute the child will recover, often with a cry, and colour will return to the face.

- **Benign paroxysmal vertigo**
  Children aged between 2 and 9 years will suddenly and for no reason look frightened, and may run to and cling on to a parent or to a piece of furniture. Older children may mention that the room appears to be spinning around. After a number of seconds this feeling and any fear goes away and the child quickly returns to normal. Children are not confused or sleepy after these attacks.

- **Simple faints**
  Also called syncopal or vaso-vagal attacks, these are very

common, particularly in teenage girls. Faints usually occur if someone has been standing in a hot room for a long time, or is unwell with a bad cold or stomach upset. Children feel dizzy, sweaty, unwell and perhaps sick, and friends comment that they look 'deathly white' before they fall. There may be some very brief jerky movements when they are on the floor. Very rarely there may be urinary incontinence (ie children may wet themselves). Recovery is usually very quick, within a few minutes. Faints are due to a very slow heart rate, and the heart rate always speeds up when someone is lying down.

- **Migraine**
  This severe type of headache is sometimes preceded by a visual aura. Although auras may also occur in epilepsy, the aura before a migraine headache lasts for longer than an epileptic aura. There is more information about auras in epilepsy in the section on *More about seizures* in Chapter 1.

- **Narcolepsy**
  Episodes of suddenly falling asleep anywhere and anytime for anything between 30 seconds and a few minutes. This condition is extremely rare in children under 14 or 15 years of age.

- **Tics and mannerisms**
  These are quite common in children and involve regular and repeated involuntary movements. Common tics include eye-blinking, head-shaking, shoulder-shrugging and finger-tapping. They are more common in boys than in girls. The movements tend to become worse when the children are teased, under stress or tired. Most children have some degree of control over them, and will eventually grow out of them.

- **Night terrors**
  These occur in children aged 4–10 years, usually between 30–90 minutes after they fall asleep. They wake suddenly looking terrified, often screaming, not recognising parents and are inconsolable. There is no jerking and children do not usually wet themselves. Within a few minutes they fall back asleep and they have no recollection of the episode the next morning. The parents are usually the ones who need reassurance!

- **Paroxysmal choreoathetosis**
  A group of very rare conditions provoked by emotional stress or sudden movement, during which older children show rather strange writhing and twisting movements of the limbs.

- **Cardiac dysrhythmias**
  Abnormalities of heart rate or rhythm.

- **Hyperventilation**
  Overbreathing, ie breathing too hard or too fast, often due to a panic attack.

- **Pseudoseizures**
  Also called pseudo-epileptic seizures or non-epileptic attacks, these are seizures which look like epileptic seizures but are not. They often have an underlying psychological cause, and are much more common in girls than in boys, and also in teenagers rather than in younger children.

The specialist at the hospital asked exactly the same questions as our GP – why the duplication?

Because obtaining as much information as possible about what actually happened to your child is of such great importance in the diagnosis of epilepsy or in the diagnosis of those other conditions which may, at first glance, appear to be epilepsy. We realise that it can be very frustrating to go over the same thing again and again, but it cannot be stressed enough just how important this information is. It is usual to think that we have remembered everything, but it can help to go over events more than once, as sometimes it helps us to remember some small detail which may seem insignificant to us but which may be very significant to the doctor. It is crucial to get the facts right and that is why different doctors will often ask exactly the same questions!

There were a lot of questions about my son's health when he was a baby. How can what happened so many years ago be relevant to making a diagnosis now?

The doctor needs a complete picture of your son's present state of health and to get this it is often necessary to go back, even as far as your pregnancy and your son's birth, in order to find out as much information as possible. This enables the doctor to put together all the pieces of the 'diagnostic jigsaw' and so make the correct diagnosis. For example, your son might have had a head injury in the past, or an illness which can affect the brain (eg meningitis), and these could be relevant to his present condition. Epilepsy can also be a symptom of many different underlying disorders, and knowing as much as possible about your son's medical history will help the doctor rule these out or decide if further tests are needed.

Apart from answering all those questions you've mentioned, what else can we expect when my daughter goes to see the specialist?

The specialist will probably want to give your daughter a careful physical examination, and perhaps (but this is unusual) take some blood for testing. You don't say how old she is, but a younger child may also have a developmental assessment to check that her physical, mental, emotional and social skills are what would be expected for her age. All these tests will provide information about her current state of health and help her specialist reach a correct diagnosis.

These tests and examinations are important, although they are rarely helpful in deciding whether or not a child's seizures are actually due to epilepsy (most children with epilepsy have normal test results). But they can help in finding if there is an underlying cause (epilepsy may be a symptom of another problem, such as a low blood level of glucose or calcium, and this would show up in a blood test), or in identifying a particular epilepsy syndrome (when information about a child's development is needed as well as information about the seizure type), or in establishing whether or not a child has another medical condition as well as epilepsy.

Your daughter may also have an EEG, or perhaps a brain scan (most children with epilepsy do not need a scan): there are sections on both these tests later in this chapter.

I do not think that my son's epilepsy diagnosis is correct. What should I do? Is it possible to get a second opinion?

You do not say whether the diagnosis was made by your GP or by a specialist. If it was your GP, then you could ask for your son to be referred to a specialist at your local hospital (in our opinion, ALL children with suspected epilepsy should be seen by a specialist). If your son is already under the care of a hospital specialist, then in the first instance you should talk over your concerns about the diagnosis with him or her. If after this discussion you are still unhappy, then it is reasonable for you to ask for another opinion. You could, for example, ask either your son's present specialist or your GP for a referral to a paediatric neurologist who specialises in the diagnosis of epilepsy in children.

These suggestions are based on the assumption that you simply want to make sure that the diagnosis is correct.

What we cannot tell from your question is whether you are instead asking for help in coming to terms with the diagnosis. Being told that your child has epilepsy is a shock, and disbelief is a common reaction. If this is the case, then we would still suggest that talking things through with your son's specialist would be a good starting point. There is also a section on *Coming to terms with epilepsy* in Chapter 5, and you might find this helpful.

EEGs

What exactly is an EEG?

Confusingly, the abbreviation EEG stands for both electroencephalograph (the EEG machine) and electroencephalogram (the recording made on the paper). Even more confusingly, many people use the two words the other way around, ie electroencephalogram for the machine and electroencephalograph for the recording. ('Encephalo' comes from the Greek word 'enkephalos' which means 'in the head'.) To avoid this problem, in this book we have kept to the abbreviation or used the terms 'EEG machine' and 'EEG recording' where appropriate.

An EEG is a test which records and measures the tiny electrical signals (sometimes called 'brainwaves') produced inside the brain. It provides a picture of the electrical activity inside the brain, whether it be the normal activity that goes on all the time or the 'out of the correct order' activity that occurs during a seizure (there is more information about this in the section on *Epilepsy and the brain* in Chapter 1).

During an EEG, small discs called electrodes are placed on the child's head. Between eight and 32 electrodes may be used, depending on the age of the child, but usually 16 or 20 electrodes are required. These electrodes pick up the brainwaves and transfer them to the EEG machine where they are amplified (enlarged). They are then displayed on a

TV screen or recorded as a trace on a roll of graph paper.

The EEG recording consists of several lines, and each line is a picture of the brainwaves being produced by a different part of the brain (determined by the placing of the electrodes). This means that the EEG can show not only what is happening, but also where in the brain it is happening.

An EEG is completely painless. The electricity goes only from the brain to the machine, not the other way around, so there is absolutely no risk of a child getting an electric shock. A routine EEG in the out-patient department of a hospital only takes from 30–90 minutes to complete (the time varies depending on the co-operation of the child – lying still is important). Parents' main complaint about EEGs is the hairwashing that is needed afterwards – the electrodes sometimes have to be stuck to the child's head with a special glue! However, it is possible for the electrodes to be held in place by other techniques, including something that looks like a rubber hairnet.

What part do EEGs play in making a diagnosis of epilepsy?

They are invaluable tools in the investigation and classification of epilepsy, providing that they are recorded carefully and interpreted correctly. (Ideally children should have their EEGs carried out in a paediatric EEG unit where the staff not only have a high standard of technical skills but are also specially trained to deal with children of all ages.) They are NOT a substitute for a clinical diagnosis (ie one based on what the doctor observes and on the information you and your child provide). EEGs should never be interpreted in isolation, but always in conjunction with what is happening clinically. In other words, they should only be used to support a clinical diagnosis of epilepsy, and to help decide what type of seizure is involved. Doctors combine the information provided by EEGs with what is known about a child's seizure type or types to help them find out if the child has a particular type of epilepsy or epilepsy syndrome (there is more information about recognising epilepsy syndromes in the section on *Types of epilepsy* in Chapter 1).

If EEGs are so useful, why shouldn't they be used on their own to confirm an epilepsy diagnosis?

Because they have their limitations as well as their uses. As almost 50% of children with epilepsy have normal EEGs between seizures, for most types of epilepsy (there are a couple of exceptions) EEGs can only confirm the diagnosis if a child actually has a seizure while the EEG is being recorded – and seizures do not usually happen to order! Other limitations are that about 10%–15% of people who do not have epilepsy have EEGs that do not look normal, and there are also a number of people who have no history of seizures but whose EEGs show epilepsy-type patterns. Add to these limitations the fact that movements (even just opening and closing the eyes, or sucking and chewing) can show up on the recording, and you can see why interpreting EEGs correctly needs so much expertise.

What sort of thing are doctors looking for on EEG recordings?

They are looking for the out-of-the-ordinary brainwave patterns (called 'discharges') which show that the electrical signals in the brain are not being sent smoothly and in the correct order. The shapes of the discharges and how frequently they occur during the recording provide information about the type of seizure. Discharges are more likely to be seen on ictal EEGs (those recorded when a seizure is actually taking place) than on interictal EEGs (those recorded between seizures). 'Ictal' comes from the Latin word 'ictus', which means a strike or sudden blow (the Latin phrase for an epileptic seizure is 'ictus epilepticus').

Figure 7 shows an example of a normal EEG recording (the outline of the head in the figure shows where the electrodes were placed). The brainwave patterns are sym-

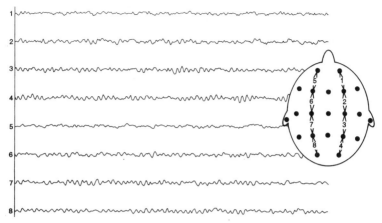

Figure 7: Normal EEG recording.

metrical and regular and show the electrical activity that goes on in the brain all the time.

By contrast, Figure 8 shows an EEG recording full of discharges. This is hypsarrhythmia, named from the Greek words 'hypsi' meaning 'aloft' and 'arhythmos' meaning 'absence of rhythm'. A good translation of hypsarrhythmia is 'mountainous chaos' as the recording is full of jumbled irregular peaks (the technical term for peaks in an EEG recording is 'spikes'). This pattern occurs in a rare type of epilepsy called infantile spasms or West syndrome which affects babies of under a year old. It is one of the few instances where an EEG recording can be used to make a definite diagnosis, as the interictal and ictal patterns are the same. However, if a child with infantile spasms responds well to treatment (something which will usually depend on the underlying cause of the syndrome) then the interictal EEG can change dramatically and go back almost to normal.

Figure 9 shows an EEG pattern called 'spike and slow

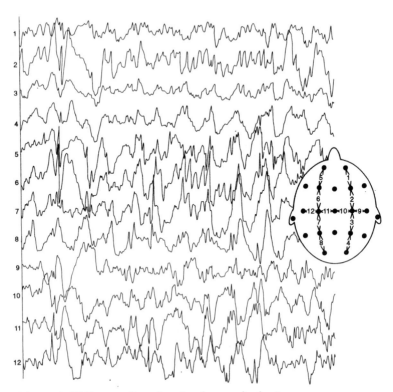

Figure 8: EEG recording showing hypsarrhythmia.

wave'. As it occurs in all the lines on the recording, it indicates a generalised seizure – an absence seizure in this particular example (there is more information about both generalised seizures and absence seizures in Chapter 1). EEGs of absence seizures typically show a pattern of three spike and slow wave discharges each second (technically this is described as 3 Hz or 3 cycles/second spike and slow wave activity). This is an ictal pattern (ie it only appears when a seizure is taking place), and between seizures the EEG pattern appears normal. If a child is thought to have absence seizures, then 99% of the time it is possible to bring

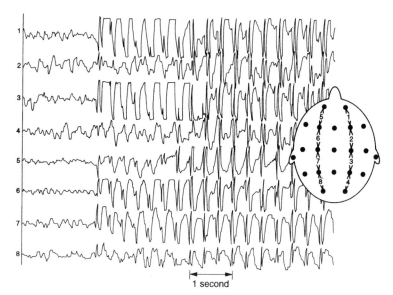

Figure 9: EEG recording of an absence seizure showing spike and slow wave pattern.

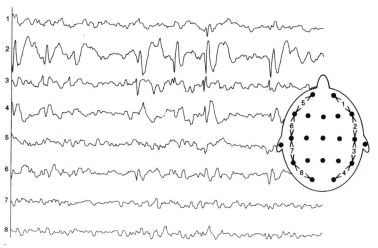

Figure 10: EEG recording of a partial seizure starting in the right side of the brain (electrodes 2 and 3).

one on by encouraging the child to hyperventilate (over-breathe, ie breathe much faster and more deeply than normal). If this is done while the EEG is being recorded, then the typical EEG pattern we have just described will be absolute confirmation of the diagnosis.

Figure 10 provides an example of why the information provided by an EEG cannot be used on its own (discussed in the answers to the previous two questions in this section). A spike and slow wave pattern appears again, but this time only on some of the lines of the recording. This pattern is both ictal and interictal, and indicates a partial seizure (in this example one starting in the right side of the brain). However, there is no way of telling from the recording whether it is a simple partial seizure or a complex one (there is more information about these types of seizure in Chapter 1). The specialist also needs to know exactly what happened to the child during a seizure in order to make a definite diagnosis. For example, if the child had some twitching on the left side of the body (the right side of the brain controls the left side of the body) but remained fully conscious, then this would suggest a simple partial seizure. If the child became confused or behaved in a strange way, then this would indicate an affected level of consciousness, and would suggest a complex partial seizure.

My teenage son had his first seizure when he was watching television. When he had his EEG they made him look at a flashing light and he had another seizure. What was the point of doing this?

To check for photosensitivity (there is more information about photosensitivity in the section *More about seizures* in Chapter 1). A diagnosis of photosensitivity was suggested by the fact that your son's first seizure occurred when he was watching television, and the stroboscope test (the flashing light used during his EEG, sometimes called a strobe) was used to confirm it. If his body jerked briefly

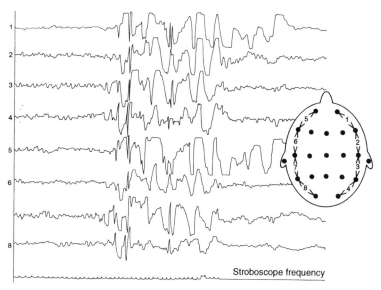

Figure 11: EEG recording showing what happens when a photo-sensitive child looks at a stroboscope.

when he was looking at the light, then he had a photo-convulsive response.

The EEG recording in Figure 11 shows what happens to the brainwaves when a photosensitive child looks at a stroboscope. The stroboscope has triggered a generalised irregular spike and slow wave discharge (these terms are explained in the answer to the previous question). The line below the EEG indicates the stroboscope frequency – in this example it is flashing 12–14 times a second (technically speaking, it has a frequency of 12–14 cycles/second or 12–14 Hz).

My 3-year-old daughter has already been to out-patients for one EEG, and now we've been told she has to have another one. Surely the results will just be the same as the first time, so why do they need to repeat it?

A routine EEG in the out-patients department of a hospital

takes somewhere between 30–90 minutes, and it does have its limitations. For example, it is quite a long time for a young child to stay still (although many children do fall asleep during the recording), so if your daughter was particularly restless it would have affected the results. A more important limitation is that it is rare for a seizure to actually occur during an EEG, and interictal EEGs (ie those recorded between seizures) often appear normal.

These problems can be solved using a variety of specialised EEG techniques (they are discussed in the rest of this section) and it may be that your daughter is going to have one of these tests next time. The results of her second EEG may well provide different and more informative results than her first one. It is quite usual for EEGs to be repeated until enough evidence has been collected for a specialist to be able to confirm a particular type of seizure or identify a specific epilepsy syndrome.

My son is very active, he only stops moving when he is asleep. He has severe learning difficulties as well as epilepsy, and I don't think we could explain to him the need to lie still during the recording. Will this stop him have an EEG when he needs one?

No, he could have what is known as a sedation EEG. This simply means that he would be given a sedative to help him relax and lie still or perhaps go to sleep while the EEG is being recorded.

I was asked to make sure that my young son stayed awake for some time before he went to the clinic for his EEG, he wasn't allowed to have his usual naps. Why wouldn't they let him sleep?

It sounds as if your son was going to have a sleep-deprived EEG, perhaps because his routine EEG had appeared normal. Reducing a child's normal or full amount of sleep can cause changes in the electrical signals in the brain (it is rare for it to provoke a seizure). These changes would not be seen in a routine EEG, but when they appear after sleep deprivation they may provide important evidence to support a diagnosis of epilepsy. Sleep deprivation also makes it more likely that your son will fall asleep naturally during the test (although it doesn't matter if he stays awake), and this is another way that more helpful information can be obtained.

Lisa fell asleep during her EEG, and the hospital staff were very pleased about this as they said it gave them extra information about her epilepsy. Please can you explain why?

There are two possible reasons. The first depends on whether or not Lisa is one of those children who only ever have seizures when they are asleep (nocturnal seizures). If she is, then the only possible chance of recording a seizure on a routine EEG is for her to sleep during the test! However, the chances of recording nocturnal seizures on a routine EEG are quite low. If Lisa's seizures are of this type then she will probably need one of the specialised EEG techniques which are more suitable for recording nocturnal seizures, and these are discussed in the answers to the next two questions.

The second and perhaps more important reason is that brainwaves change dramatically during sleep (this happens to everyone, not just people with epilepsy). Research has shown that sleep can activate or unmask out-of-the-ordinary brainwave patterns (discharges). In particular, being asleep can enhance the interictal patterns on the EEG recording (ie make the brainwave patterns between seizures more obvious), which means that they provide more information and give the specialist extra clues which will help in making a diagnosis of a particular type of seizure or epilepsy syndrome. From this point of view, the most important time is the initial stage of falling asleep, when the child is just 'drifting off', as it is during this period that the discharges are most likely to be recorded. Lisa will not need to have a seizure during the recording for this activity to show up on her EEG.

My son only ever has seizures in his sleep, so the specialist wants him to have a night-time EEG. Does he have to stay in hospital for this, or can he have it at home?

It will depend on the facilities available at your local hospital. A night-time EEG can be carried out at home using a technique called ambulatory monitoring (described in the answer to the next question). However, the equipment needed for this is only available at a few hospitals – if your local hospital is not one of them, then he will have to stay there overnight to have the test.

What is ambulatory monitoring?

Ambulatory monitoring is a portable type of EEG – it literally means 'EEG monitoring while walking about' (from the Latin word 'ambulare' meaning 'to walk'). It allows a child's brainwaves to be recorded continuously over anything from several hours to a few days, a much longer period of time than a routine EEG. The aim is to collect as much evidence as possible to help with the diagnosis. The longer time period makes it more likely that a seizure will be recorded, and the portable equipment means that the test is taking place during the child's normal everyday activities, rather than in the strange surroundings of a hospital. It is particularly useful for those children who have only nocturnal (sleep) seizures.

In ambulatory monitoring, electrodes are attached to the child's head just as in a routine EEG. The electrodes are then connected to a recorder which is about the size of a personal cassette player and which is worn in just the same way, either around the waist or over the shoulder. The brainwaves are continuously recorded onto the cassette in the recorder. At the end of the test, the tape from the cassette is analysed using specialised computer equipment. This converts the magnetic signals on the tape back to a standard EEG tracing, ready to be interpreted by a specialist in the usual way.

The specialist isn't sure that my daughter has epilepsy, he thinks there may be some other reason for her seizures. He wants to video her the next time she has an EEG. How will this help him decide if she has epilepsy or not?

The test your daughter is going to have is called video-telemetry (telemetry literally means 'measurement from a distance'). It uses a video camera linked to an EEG machine, which will allow simultaneous recording of what your daughter is doing and the electrical activity in her brain (the brainwaves). When the videotape is played back, one half of the screen will show your daughter and the other half her EEG recording (which explains the alternative name for this test – 'split screen EEG'). This means that the clinical evidence (what is actually happening to your daughter) and the electrical evidence (the EEG recording) can be looked at together.

Videotelemetry is very helpful in making an accurate diagnosis of epilepsy. There are a number of other conditions which are not epilepsy but which can produce episodes or attacks which may resemble or look like an epileptic seizure (they were discussed in the previous section of this chapter). It is also possible for a child to have epilepsy but for a routine EEG to look normal. The direct comparison of a seizure and its EEG that videotelemetry allows provides a solution for these diagnostic problems. If the videocamera records your daughter having one of her attacks but the EEG is normal, then it is highly likely (but not impossible) that she does not have epilepsy and the specialist knows to look for another cause for her condition. If instead the EEG shows a pattern typical of epilepsy, then the diagnosis of epilepsy is confirmed.

Another advantage of videotelemetry is that a child can be observed over periods of several hours (or even several days if it is thought necessary) which means that it is more likely that a seizure will be recorded. The camera acts as the eyewitness (the importance of an accurate eyewitness account was also discussed in the previous section of this chapter) with the added advantage of the simultaneous EEG recording. This makes it a very useful tool in the classification of epilepsy, as well as in accurate diagnosis. Unfortunately the equipment needed is extremely expensive, and so the test is only available in a limited number of hospitals. It is also more often used in adults (and in particular in those who are being considered for a surgical treatment for their epilepsy) than in children.

SCANS

What is a brain scan?

A painless and completely harmless way of producing clear and detailed pictures of the brain. The two main types are CT scanning and MRI.

A CT scan uses x-rays to produce images of the brain which are then fed into a computer. The computer reconstructs these images into 'slices' – pictures of cross-sections of the brain. When these pictures are viewed in the correct order, they build up a picture of the whole brain. CT stands for computed or computerised tomography (tomography comes from two Greek words – 'tomos' meaning 'a slice' and 'graphein' meaning 'to draw'). It is also referred to as CAT scanning (computer assisted tomography or computerised axial tomography).

Instead of x-rays, MRI uses magnetism: MRI stands for magnetic resonance imaging. The pictures of the brain it produces are similar to those produced by CT scanning, but are much more detailed. For example, a CT scan is an appropriate initial investigation to exclude the possibility of a brain tumour (a very rare cause of epilepsy in children, discussed at the end of this section). But CT scans are less sensitive than MRI in detecting very small brain lesions (abnormalities), particularly within the frontal and temporal lobes (the lobes of the brain are shown in Figure 2 in Chapter 1).

A child having a brain scan will notice little difference between the two types – they both involve lying still within a hollow cylinder at the centre of the scanning machine. Children who have difficulty in lying still or who are very frightened by the machine (MRI machines can be very noisy) may be given a sedative or even a quick general anaesthetic.

CT scanning and MRI both show the structure of the brain. Newer type of scans called SPECT scanning (SPECT stands for single photon emission computerised tomography) and PET scanning (PET stands for positron emission tomography) also provide information about how the brain is functioning. In the future these types of scan may prove helpful in understanding the classification and causes of epilepsy, but at present their use is limited to a few specialised centres.

Should every child with epilepsy have a brain scan?

No, as most children with epilepsy do not require one. For example, children with primary idiopathic generalised epilepsies (eg typical absence epilepsy or juvenile myoclonic epilepsy) or with some benign partial epilepsies do not routinely require a scan (there is a section on *Types of epilepsy* in Chapter 1).

A scan can be useful if there is a possibility that a child's epilepsy has been caused by something actually going wrong with the structure of the brain – perhaps the brain never developed properly, or has been injured or damaged, or has been affected in some other way. The specialist will probably already be suspicious that this may have happened, as there will be other indications as well as epilepsy. For example, the child may have other neurological abnormalities or disorders (ie other problems affecting the brain or nervous system) or show signs of developmental problems (ie if the child's physical, mental, emotional and social skills do not seem to be developing as they should).

Scans are more usually performed to try to find an underlying cause for epilepsy in children under a year old who have either partial seizures, myoclonic seizures or infantile spasms (again see the section on *Types of epilepsy* in Chapter 1 for more information about these). Other children who may need a scan are those whose seizures return without explanation following an initial period of good control with anti-epileptic drugs.

The specialist said the scans were fine, does this mean that my son doesn't have epilepsy?

No, not necessarily, as the majority of children with epilepsy have normal scans. Scans cannot be used to diagnose epilepsy, but they may be helpful in revealing an underlying cause, or confirming that no such cause exists. In almost 75% of all children diagnosed as having epilepsy, no specific cause for it will be found (there is more about this in the section on *Possible causes* in Chapter 1).

A brain scan may sometimes have to be repeated, although fortunately this is a rare occurrence. A repeat scan is more likely to be necessary for those children whose seizure type has changed or in whom seizure control is poor, and whose first scan was a CT scan done many years ago. Any repeat brain scan will almost certainly be the more detailed MRI scan.

I have read in the paper that MRI scans can diagnose epilepsy. Is this true? We haven't got an MRI scanner near us, so should we put pressure on our doctor to send our daughter elsewhere for one?

The diagnosis of epilepsy is always a clinical diagnosis (see the section on *How do they know it's epilepsy?* earlier in this chapter for the reasons). MRI (magnetic resonance imaging) therefore cannot diagnose epilepsy. However, it is a useful investigation in some groups of children with epilepsy which may reveal an underlying cause for seizures.

The decision to carry out MRI depends upon the clinical evidence (ie what your doctor has observed about your daughter and the information you have provided about her seizures). Not every child who has epilepsy needs such a scan, and your daughter may well be among this group. We would suggest that you arrange to talk it through with your doctor to find out if your daughter really needs MRI. This would be preferable to putting on pressure for what may be an unnecessary test.

I'm frightened that my daughter's epilepsy means that she may have a brain tumor. She is going to have a scan – does this mean her specialist thinks so too?

Not necessarily. Scans can show whether or not someone has a brain tumor, but they can also show other things as well, so the fact that she is going to have a scan does not automatically mean that her specialist suspects a tumor. It is important to remember that in children brain tumours are very rarely a cause of epilepsy – only 1%–2% of all epilepsy in all children is caused by such a tumour. As we do not know the details of your daughter's epilepsy, we would suggest that you talk your fears over with the specialist, who will be able to explain exactly why your daughter is to have her scan.

CHAPTER 3

Treatment

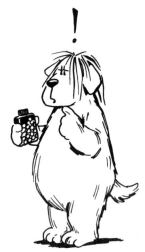

INTRODUCTION

The terms 'anti-epileptic' and 'anti-convulsant' are often used interchangeably by doctors when they are talking about epilepsy treatments. Both terms mean exactly the same thing. You may also hear doctors talking about a 'drug', 'treatment', 'therapy' or 'medication': once again these are all interchangeable terms. In this book we have decided to use the expression 'anti-epileptic drug', but this is just our personal choice, and your child's doctor may prefer another term. Much of this chapter is about these anti-epileptic drugs, as they are the most usual treatment for epilepsy. But we also consider epilepsy surgery, and look at what place (if any) the complementary therapies have in the care of children with epilepsy.

DOES TREATMENT WORK?

How easy is epilepsy to control?

As you are probably aware, there are many different types of epileptic seizure and many different types of epilepsy (they are discussed in the section on *Types of epilepsy* in Chapter 1). Fortunately, most types of seizure and most types of epilepsy are fairly easy to control with treatment. This includes being able to stop the seizures for up to two or more years. Overall, about 70%–75% of children with epilepsy will have their seizures controlled completely with one anti-epileptic drug. In another 5%–10% of children the epilepsy will be controlled, but only by using a combination of two drugs.

In the remaining 15%–25% of children epilepsy will never be fully controlled. It is in this group that anti-epileptic drugs may need to be changed every few months or even every few weeks, to try to find the most suitable drug or drugs (ie those which can control as many seizures as possible and without causing side-effects). Unfortunately, this may take some time – even many months – to achieve. Occasionally seizures can be controlled for several months but then, for a number of reasons, this control can be lost and the seizures may start again. This could happen either because the child is not taking the anti-epileptic drugs as prescribed, or because a larger dose may be needed. It may be the result of another illness (discussed in the section on *Practical aspects of drug treatment* later in this chapter) or it may simply be a feature of that particular type of epilepsy. In children, the seizure types that are more difficult to control are myoclonic, atonic, tonic and partial seizures; the difficult to control epilepsies or epilepsy syndromes are infantile spasms (also called West syndrome), Lennox-Gastaut syndrome, severe myoclonic epilepsy and myoclonic astatic epilepsy.

Our daughter's seizures are very difficult to control and drug after drug has been used. The hospital doctor just seems to be adding one drug to another. Is it right that she should be taking four anti-epileptic drugs?

In the answer to the previous question we mentioned that seizures can be controlled with a single anti-epileptic drug in about 70%–75% of all children with epilepsy. Unfortunately, this statistic also means that between 25% and 30% of children will not have their seizures controlled by just one drug. Sometimes adding another drug (so that the child is taking two) will then control the seizures – whichever two drugs are used will be chosen because they work well together. It is very rare for three anti-epileptic drugs to work where two have not, and this should be avoided whenever possible.

No child should be treated with four anti-epileptic drugs, not only because four drugs will be ineffective and unhelpful, but also because there will be an increased chance of side-effects. It is very important that you talk to your daughter's hospital doctor about your concerns, and we would recommend that you arrange to do this as soon as possible.

Does epilepsy ever just go away?

Yes, epilepsy does sometimes 'go away' of its own accord. The technical term for this is 'spontaneous remission'. It means that the child will stop having seizures and will be able to stop taking anti-epileptic drugs. However, it only happens in certain types of epilepsy and it is not that easy to predict, or even to know exactly when the epilepsy has 'gone away'.

Two types of epilepsy where the seizures usually do stop of their own accord are typical absence epilepsy of childhood and BREC (benign rolandic epilepsy of childhood). Seizures will stop by puberty in about 70%–75% of children with typical absence epilepsy. In the case of BREC it is thought that all seizures will eventually stop in every child that has it and the drugs used to treat it can then be withdrawn. This is also often around puberty (13–16 years of age), but may be earlier.

Can epilepsy treatment ever be stopped?

Sometimes. As doctors cannot predict exactly when seizures will stop and the epilepsy will have gone into spontaneous remission, it is difficult to know for how long anti-epileptic drugs should be taken before they can be withdrawn. Most doctors would advise that if a child has been receiving treatment and has had no seizures for two or sometimes three years, then the drug can be gradually withdrawn. Any anti-epileptic drug must be withdrawn or reduced gradually over at least 6–8 weeks (and sometimes longer) before stopping it altogether. Stopping taking treatment suddenly can be dangerous and could lead to a condition called status epilepticus (an emergency which is discussed further in Chapter 4).

There is a slight chance that a child's seizures will return after treatment is stopped, but this will depend on the type of seizures and the type of epilepsy that the child has had in the past. If it does happen it usually does so within a few weeks or months of the drug being withdrawn, but it may not happen for one or even more years. If the seizures do return, they are likely to be of the same type as those that occurred before.

ANTI-EPILEPTIC DRUGS

Why do anti-epileptic drugs have two names?

It is not just anti-epileptic drugs which have two names – nearly all drugs do. The first is the generic (the chemical or scientific) name, which is given to the drug when it is first developed. The second is the brand (or trade) name, which is decided by the pharmaceutical company which makes the drug. Sometimes a drug has more than one brand name, which means that it is produced by more than one company, each of which has given it a different brand name. Generic names are usually written with a small first letter and brand names with a capital first letter.

It can be useful to know the generic names of your child's anti-epileptic drugs as well as the brand names, particularly if you are going abroad (there is more information about obtaining drugs overseas in the section on *Medical care abroad* in Chapter 8). Brand names can vary from country to country, but the generic names of drugs are internationally standardised and will be recognised by pharmacists in any part of the world where the drug is available. Generic names must, by law, be printed somewhere on the original container (although they may appear in very small print). The table in Figure 12 lists the brand and generic names of the most-commonly used anti-epileptic drugs.

The whole subject of drug names is further complicated by the age of the drugs (ie how long it has been since a drug was first produced). Pharmaceutical companies patent the drugs they develop, and so newer drugs (ie those still under patent protection) are only available as the brand name product (they still have a generic name, but they cannot be sold as a generic product). On the other hand, drugs which have been available for a very long time (eg phenobarbitone, which first became available in 1912) may only be available under their generic names!

This seems a good place to mention two other very old drugs which are available only as generic products, both of which are still in occasional use today. The first is paraldehyde which is used ONLY to stop prolonged seizures or convulsions including status epilepticus (there is a section on *Status epilepticus* in Chapter 4). It is effective but it has a strong smell which some people may find a little unpleasant. The second drug is called bromide, and it was in fact the first ever drug used to treat epilepsy (it was discovered in

BRAND NAME	GENERIC NAME
Ativan	lorazepam
Convulex	valproic acid
Diamox	acetazolamide
Diazemuls	diazepam
Emeside	ethosuximide
Epanutin	phenytoin
Epilim	sodium valproate
Epilim Chrono	sodium valproate
Frisium	clobazam
Lamictal	lamotrigine
Mogadon	nitrazepam
Mysoline	primidone
Neurontin	gabapentin
Nootropil	piracetam
Rivotril	clonazepam
Sabril	vigabatrin
Stesolid	diazepam (as a rectal tube only)
Tegretol	carbamazepine
Tegretol Retard	carbamazepine
Topamax	topiramate
Valium	diazepam
Zarontin	ethosuximide

Figure 12: Brand and generic names of anti-epileptic drugs.

1880). It has a number of side-effects, some of which may be very unpleasant, and it is very rarely used – only in a few specialist epilepsy centres and in very specialised circumstances.

Are there any real differences between branded drugs and their generic equivalents?

The actual drug is the same, whether it be a branded version or a generic one, and both versions should have the same effect in controlling seizures. It is important to remember this, as the products may look very different. For example, the generic version of a particular drug may be available only as a plain white tablet or capsule or as an unflavoured liquid, while the branded product may be a coloured tablet or capsule or a more pleasantly-flavoured liquid.

Occasionally there may be a difference between the generic and the branded product in the way in which the tablet, capsule or liquid has been manufactured. Because of this, if a prescription is changed from the generic drug to the brand name drug (or vice versa), then sometimes the frequency of seizures may change (either increase or decrease) or some side-effects may develop. It is therefore important to continue with whichever version was first prescribed – it does not matter whether this was the generic drug or the branded drug, just as long as all future prescriptions use the same name.

Generic drugs are usually less expensive than branded drugs, so doctors are often encouraged to prescribe a generic version, if one is available, to keep National Health Service costs down. This price difference will not matter to you or your child as people with epilepsy do not have to pay NHS prescription charges (information on prescription charge exemption is in the section on *Finance* in Chapter 7).

I went to my first epilepsy group meeting the other day, and people there were talking about the different types of drugs. I was surprised to learn that the same drug can be available in lots of different forms – as a tablet or a capsule or a liquid and so on. Why?

Most of the anti-epileptic drugs come in two or three different forms (also called preparations, formulations or formats). The choice of formulations means that it should be possible for everyone to find a version of their anti-epileptic drug which is both convenient and easy to swallow. For example, a young child who has difficulty swallowing a whole tablet may find it easier to take a liquid version of the same drug, while an older child who takes a midday dose at school might prefer tablets or capsules as they are easier to carry. There are four common formulations of anti-epileptic drugs.

- **Tablets**
  Also called pills, these can either be swallowed whole, chewed or crushed. Others can be dissolved in water or fruit juice which is then drunk (these tablets are called dispersible tablets). Some tablets have a special coating: these are known as 'enteric-coated' tablets. The reason for this is that some anti-epileptic drugs can irritate the stomach which can produce some discomfort, including diarrhoea. The enteric coating reduces the chance of this happening ('enteric' comes from the Greek word 'enteron' which means gut or intestine).

- **Capsules**
  These can either be swallowed whole or sometimes (depending on the particular anti-epileptic drug) a capsule can be opened up and the contents inside emptied out and given to a child with a favourite fruit juice or food.

- **Liquids**
  These are often flavoured, and some are available in sugar-free formulations to protect children's teeth.

- **Powders**
  These are taken dissolved in water, fruit juice or even milk.

Exactly which of these will be available will depend on the particular drug, as not all anti-epileptic drugs are available in all formulations. For example, some drugs will not be available as capsules, while others will not be available as a powder. Your doctor will know what formulations are available for any particular anti-epileptic drug that your child is prescribed. It is important to realise that, generally speaking, the drug will do the same job just as effectively no matter what the formulation.

The British Epilepsy Association (address in Appendix 1) produces a colour poster showing the shapes and colours of the most commonly-prescribed tablets and capsules. The poster also includes other information about these drugs, such as their brand and generic names, the packaging they come in, and the other formulations available.

Are all anti-epileptic drugs designed to be swallowed or can they be given in other ways?

Regular anti-epileptic medication is always given orally (by mouth) and is designed to be swallowed. However, other ways of giving some of the drugs can be used in special circumstances, for example in an emergency. One formulation of one particular anti-epileptic drug is a solution designed to be given into the rectum (the back passage, also referred to as the anus). The generic name of this drug is diazepam, the brand name is Stesolid and it comes in a small tube with a nozzle which is inserted into a child's rectum.

Stesolid is not used on a regular, daily basis but is only given in an emergency when a child has a seizure which lasts for more than a few minutes. Clearly a drug cannot be given by mouth during a seizure as the child will be unable to swallow, but giving the drug into the rectum is effective because it is well absorbed into the blood stream from there. Parents only need to learn when and how to use Stesolid if their child has epilepsy which is firstly difficult to control and secondly likely to lead to frequent and long seizures.

The other anti-epileptic drug which is available in a rectal solution is paraldehyde, which is NEVER given by mouth. Paraldehyde is only used to stop prolonged seizures and never on a regular daily basis.

There are also some anti-epileptic drugs which can be given by injection either intramuscularly (into a muscle) or intravenously (into a vein). These injections are usually only given in hospital, again in an emergency situation to try and stop a child's seizure which has gone on for too long.

Can you reassure me that the newer anti-epileptic drugs are really safe for children to take?

This is a little difficult to answer, but we would say yes – probably! Not only are all new anti-epileptic drugs thoroughly tested, they are all first used for adults with epilepsy before being used for children. Because of this, the particular 'licence' (the permit which sets out how a drug should be prescribed) is different for children and adults. The licence only becomes the same for both groups when a drug has been around and available for many years.

At the moment there is a lot of research going on into finding and manufacturing new anti-epileptic drugs for children. The three most recent ones which have been used are vigabatrin (Sabril), lamotrigine (Lamictal) and gabapentin (Neurontin). Many more drugs are currently being researched and developed and will probably become available in the next 3–5 years.

There is a big difference between the 'older' and 'newer' anti-epileptic drugs. The newer ones have been designed and made specifically to treat epilepsy, whereas the older ones were often first intended for the treatment of other conditions, but then also proved useful as anti-epileptics. This targeting of the newer drugs means that they tend to have fewer serious side-effects than the older drugs, and could therefore in one sense be said to be 'safer'. However, because they are new and have not been around for all that long, not a lot is known about their longer-term effects.

Our son's specialist has suggested that steroids may be helpful

in treating his epilepsy. We have heard a lot of bad things about steroids – are they safe and should we let our son have them?

We should first make it clear that the steroids we are talking about here are not the same as those abused by a few athletes to 'build up' their muscles or improve their performance. Those are anabolic steroids, and we are concerned with a type called corticosteroids. Confusion can arise because both types are referred to by the abbreviation 'steroids'.

It is difficult to answer your question completely as we do not know the sort of epileptic seizure and type of epilepsy that your son has. However, steroids are sometimes (but usually only rarely) prescribed for children who have particular types of seizures which occur many times a day. These include infantile spasms (also called West syndrome), myoclonic seizures and atonic seizures (you will find more information about these in the sections on *Types of epilepsy* and *More about seizures* in Chapter 1).

The most commonly used steroids are prednisolone (also called prednisone) and ACTH (which stands for adrenocorticotrophic hormone). Betamethasone is a less commonly used steroid. Prednisolone and betamethasone are given by mouth, and ACTH only by an injection (into the muscles of the buttocks or thighs). We do not know why steroids work – and they do not always stop the seizures. Even if the seizures are controlled, they may return as soon as the steroid treatment is stopped.

You are quite right in asking about their side-effects as these are common and may be serious. These side-effects are more commonly seen with ACTH than with prednisolone or betamethasone. Particularly dangerous ones include high blood pressure and reducing the body's defences in fighting infections. Children nearly always put on weight and become irritable and upset when taking steroids. Because of these possibly serious side-effects, and the fact that there are newer and safer anti-epileptic drugs, steroids are now only very rarely prescribed for these difficult seizure types and epilepsies. We would suggest that you should discuss this further with your son's specialist.

SIDE-EFFECTS

Do all the anti-epileptic drugs have side-effects?

All drugs can cause side-effects, even the ones we take for granted such as aspirin and paracetamol, and this is also true for the anti-epileptic drugs. The 'older' anti-epileptic drugs such as phenobarbitone and phenytoin (both of which were in use before World War II) usually cause more frequent and more severe side-effects than the 'newer' ones such as vigabatrin, lamotrigine and gabapentin (all of which have come into use within the last 10 years). Sodium valproate and carbamazepine (drugs first used in the 1960s and 1970s) usually have fewer side-effects than the 'older' drugs but may have one or two more than the 'newer' ones!

What are the side-effects? Is there anything that makes them more likely to happen?

Because the anti-epileptic drugs work on or act in the brain (to control the seizures, which start in the brain), they may also cause side-effects which affect the brain. Such side-effects may include drowsiness, lethargy (a feeling of tiredness), dizziness, nausea (feeling sick), a change in appetite (usually, but not always, an increase) and sometimes difficulties with co-ordination, mood or behaviour. Some drugs can be associated with rare but serious side-effects which may affect the skin, liver or bone marrow (the bone marrow is an essential organ of the body which is important in producing all the different blood cells).

Side-effects are more likely to occur if an anti-epileptic drug is started at a high dose and increased too rapidly. They are also more common when a child is taking two or more anti-epileptic drugs at the same time. Fortunately most children need only take one or, occasionally, two anti-epileptic drugs to control their seizures. Taking three or more drugs hardly ever results in better seizure control, but nearly always causes more side-effects.

How can we know when something is a side-effect of his drugs and not a new or a different illness?

It is important to ask your child's doctor (either the GP or the hospital specialist) about any possible side-effects, how common or rare they are likely to be, and what you should look out for. Some doctors provide written information sheets on the anti-epileptic drugs, and these will include details on any possible side-effects and how to recognise them.

Side-effects may be either easy or difficult to recognise – depending, obviously, on what the side-effect is and on the child being affected by it. For example, if the side-effect is a skin rash or some loss of hair then it will be easier to recognise than if it is only a feeling of sickness (nausea) or a loss of appetite. It may be harder still to recognise side-effects in very young children or in children who have learning or communication difficulties: they may be unable to describe what is happening to them and how they are feeling. In these circumstances it can occasionally be helpful to measure the exact amount of anti-epileptic drug in the blood to see whether or not the child is getting too much of it.

Should all children have regular blood tests to monitor their drug treatment?

No, this is not necessary. A blood test can be used to measure the precise amount of an anti-epileptic drug in a child's blood, but it is important to realise that the vast majority of children taking such drugs do not need to have these blood levels measured. The levels only need to be measured in the following situations:

- if the doctor thinks that a child is not taking or is not being given the drug(s);
- if a child has an episode of status epilepticus (there is a section on *Status epilepticus* in Chapter 4);
- if a child is being treated with phenytoin, as the metabolism (breakdown) of this drug in the body is complicated, particularly in young children;
- if a child has moderate to severe learning or language difficulties and so may not be able to either complain of or describe possible side-effects.

I have been told that anti-epileptic drugs can cause behaviour problems. Is this true?

Many parents have said that their children's behaviour changed after epilepsy was diagnosed and treatment started. These changes may have been seen both at home and at school, and a child may be described as having become 'hyperactive', 'difficult', 'moody or irritable' or even 'disturbed'. It can be difficult to decide what has caused these changes, as there are at least five common reasons.

1 It may be due to the emotional and psychological consequences on your child (and on you) of being given the diagnosis of epilepsy. Brothers, sisters, school friends and teachers may all react differently when a diagnosis of epilepsy has been made. This may upset your child and lead, understandably, to some difficult behaviour. (Chapter 5 on *Feelings, families and friends* explores this subject further.)

2 It may be due to the fact that it was going to happen anyway! It is important to understand that a child's brain is continually developing from birth to 10–12 years. Because of this, not only may a child's epilepsy change, but also learning ability and behaviour. What may have been a normal pattern of learning and behaviour at the

age of 4 or 5 may have changed considerably by the age of 7, 8 or 9. This might have nothing at all to do with either the frequency of the epileptic seizures or the drugs used to treat the epilepsy.

3 It may be because of frequent seizures or – rarely – because a child may be experiencing very frequent abnormal electrical activity in the brain which can only be detected by carrying out an EEG, and often only by a specialised type of EEG (there is a section on *EEGs* in Chapter 2).

4 It may be a side-effect of an anti-epileptic drug, particularly if it was started in too large a dose, or the dose was increased too quickly.

5 Any combination of reasons 1, 2, 3 and 4 as described above!

A final point: some people think that children and adults who have epilepsy have a 'different' personality, including different, even difficult behaviour, just because they have epilepsy. This is simply NOT true.

If the drugs seem to be causing side-effects, should we just stop our daughter taking them?

No, this would be a very dangerous thing to do. It is very important that a child's anti-epileptic drug or drugs are never stopped abruptly – even if you think that the drug is not working or is causing side-effects. If an anti-epileptic drug is stopped suddenly it may cause a very prolonged seizure or series of seizures called status epilepticus. This is a medical emergency and may sometimes cause serious problems (it is discussed in more detail in Chapter 4). The most common cause of status epilepticus in all people with epilepsy (whatever their age) is suddenly stopping their drug treatment. Any anti-epileptic drug must be withdrawn or reduced gradually, before stopping it altogether, and this process should take at least 6–8 weeks. The ONLY situation in which an anti-epileptic drug can be stopped suddenly is if the child is an in-patient on a hospital ward.

None of the drugs that have been used to treat our son's epilepsy have worked and the side-effects of some of them have made him unwell. Should we ask our doctor about not using any drugs at all for a time?

There are a very small number of children in whom anti-epileptic drugs just do not work and unfortunately it does sound as if your son may be one of them. You are also quite right in saying that some of these drugs can have unpleasant side-effects. It is entirely reasonable for you to think that there is thus no point in using any of them. However, you need to remember that your son's epilepsy could in fact be much worse if he takes no treatment at all. On the other hand, it is also possible that on no treatment his seizures will be no different and he may feel better. If you would like to take your son off his drugs then you must discuss this with his doctor first and the drugs MUST be stopped gradually. Anti-epileptic drugs must be withdrawn gradually over at least 6–8 weeks (and sometimes longer) before stopping them altogether. Stopping taking treatment suddenly can be dangerous and could lead to a condition called status epilepticus (an emergency which is discussed further in Chapter 4).

PRACTICAL ASPECTS OF DRUG TREATMENT

My son went 10 days without having a seizure, then he caught some bug that was going around at school, became ill and his seizures came back. Why did they start up again – was it anything to do with him being ill?

Quite possibly. Children with epilepsy often have periods of remission from their seizures such as you have described. If seizures return during an illness it is possible that an increase in body temperature (a fever) may well be the triggering factor. If your son had gastrointestinal or metabolic problems (causing diarrhoea or vomiting), then these may have reduced the amount of anti-epileptic drug absorbed from his stomach and gut. This reduced absorption would in turn have resulted in reduced efficacy, meaning that his drugs would not have been working as well as usual, and because of this further seizures could occur. Another reason for a drug not working as well during an infection or illness is that it may be metabolised (broken down) more quickly by the body, which again reduces its effect.

Obviously it is not uncommon for children to have a 'tummy-bug' or gastroenteritis, with diarrhoea and vomiting. If a child with epilepsy vomits within one or two hours of taking a dose of an anti-epileptic drug, then the dose can be repeated. If vomiting occurs three or more hours after having taken a dose, then the drug will already have absorbed from the stomach into the blood stream and there will be no need to repeat that dose.

Anna's doctor told us that we have to give her the medicine twice a day. We thought it would help us to remember that she has to take it if we give it to her when she gets up in the morning and when she goes to bed at night. Will this be all right?

It will depend on her getting-up time and her bedtime! Strictly speaking, giving a drug twice a day means giving it every 12 hours. Although it is a good idea to try and give her the medicine at 10–12 hour intervals, this does not mean using a stopwatch to ensure that it is given to the precise minute or second. For example, her first dose could be given BETWEEN 7.00 am and 8.00 am and her second dose could be given BETWEEN 7.00 pm and 8.00 pm. If her usual bedtime is around 8.00 pm, then her evening dose could be given just before she goes to bed; if her bedtime is later, at 9.00 pm or 10.00 pm, then it would still be a good idea to give her the medicine no later than 8.30 pm or 9.00 pm.

Occasionally doctors do not make it absolutely clear as to how many times a day the tablets or medicines should be taken. Fortunately most only need to be taken twice a day. A very few anti-epileptic drugs can be taken once a day, whilst a couple of others have to be given three times a day. It is obviously important for parents to ask the doctor how many times a day a child's particular anti-epileptic drug must be given. If a medicine is to be given three times a day, then it can be a little difficult to plan the timing of the different doses, and it is useful to work backwards from the child's normal bedtime. For example, if bedtime is 8.00 pm, then a possible routine could be to give the first dose of the day between 7.00 am and 8.00 am, the second between 1.00 pm and 2.00 pm, and the third and last dose between 7.00 pm and 8.00 pm. This may mean asking the child's teachers to give the midday dose at school (there is more information about schools' policies on this in the section on *Teaching the teachers* in Chapter 6). If the child's bedtime is later, perhaps around 10.00 pm, then the routine could be to give the first dose between 7.00 am and 8.00 am, the second between 3.00 pm and 4.00 pm (as soon as the child comes back from school) and the third dose between 9.30 pm and 10.00 pm.

We are a rather absent-minded family and although I do try to remember to make sure that my son takes his anti-epileptic drugs when he should, I know that one of these days I'm going to forget and he's going to miss a dose. Is this going to be very important?

Not if it only happens occasionally. It does not usually matter if one or two doses of an anti-epileptic drug are 'missed' or forgotten. As a general rule, if a dose is missed or forgotten but within the next three or four hours someone remembers that it should have been given, then it can be given safely. If you remember the missed dose only five or more hours after it should have been given, then do not give it. Never, ever, 'double up' any dose because of a previously missed dose. This applies whether the child is taking one, two or three anti-epileptic drugs.

As you know that you have a problem with remembering your son's medication (and you are not alone – it is a very common problem), perhaps you could consider devising some system to help you remember. You do not say how old your son is, but perhaps he is old enough to contribute some ideas for a reminder system, or to remind you himself when his drugs are due, or even to start taking charge of his own treatment. You could also consider buying a 'pill reminder', as discussed in the answer to the next question.

How do 'pill reminders' work?

Pill reminders are a practical solution to the very common problem of forgetting to take medication at the right time. Basically they are containers for drugs which enable someone to have an adequate supply of their medication handy (particularly if away from home, eg at school) and also to check immediately (by looking at the divisions in the container) whether or not the appropriate dose has been taken. They vary in design, size and sophistication: your pharmacist should be able to show you what is currently available and help you select the most appropriate version. Some of the latest models have a built-in alarm which sounds to remind you that it is time for a tablet, while others even carry a small water supply to help with swallowing it.

We've been asked to keep a record of all our daughter's seizures and to bring it with us the next time we come to the hospital. This came up just as we were leaving the clinic so I didn't have time to ask why or exactly what they wanted to know. Please could you explain?

Parents are often asked to keep a 'diary' of their child's seizures between clinic visits, as this can provide very useful and important information for the doctor. Keeping such a diary will also save you having to try to remember all the

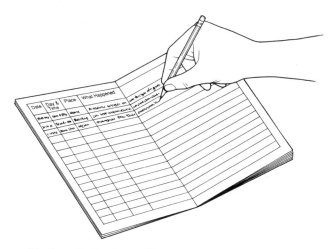

Figure 13: A typical seizure diary.

details of your daughter's seizures the next time you go to the clinic! The doctor will ask to look at the seizure diary on your next clinic visit, and will use it to assess your daughter's response to her anti-epileptic drugs (because of this, it is important that you remember to take the diary with you).

You will need to record when, where and at what time a seizure occurred, how many occurred on a single day, and what precisely happened during the seizure. You could also record any other details which you think might be important, such as any missed doses of her drugs. Some of the pharmaceutical companies which manufacture anti-epileptic drugs produce free diaries (a typical example is shown in Figure 13) and your doctor should be able to provide you with one of these, or tell you where to obtain one. However, an ordinary notebook or exercise book will do just as well.

What is the best age for our son to start taking responsibility for his own drugs?

We cannot give you a definite answer, as obviously the

'best' age will be different for every child. All children are individuals, with different attitudes and capabilities – and different types of epilepsy. We feel that it is reasonable to expect a child to start taking care of his or her own medication at an age when the parents feel that the child is sufficiently reliable and sensible. Only you can know your son well enough to judge whether or not he has reached such an age.

Often the first place outside the home where children take responsibility for their own treatment is at school, and there is a question about this in the section on *Teaching the teachers* in Chapter 6.

Recently our daughter keeps forgetting to take her medication, in fact sometimes she just refuses to take it, whatever we say. We find this extremely worrying, what on earth can we do?

Your daughter's behaviour is not unusual, not that that makes it any the less worrying for you. Non-compliance with treatment (refusing, failing or 'forgetting' to take medication) is very common in young people with epilepsy. This refusal or forgetfulness may arise from a lack of understanding about the need to take medication regularly, or it may reflect a young person's inability to accept that he or she has epilepsy – in this way it is a denial of having the condition.

Young people with epilepsy need to take over the responsibility for their own condition and with most children this usually happens gradually. Children must be given responsibility for taking their own medication, and it is important for you to show your daughter that you have trust and confidence in her ability to take care of herself (easier said than done). However, young people need to know exactly why they must take medication and parents are not always the best people to deal with this issue, especially during the rebellious stages of adolescence where anything a parent says is ignored or contradicted. Information and advice may be more acceptable if it comes from a very close friend or even another member of the family such as an uncle, aunt or grandparent.

Not wanting to take medication may also be due to some of the side-effects of the drug(s). This is particularly important for some teenage girls who are taking sodium valproate, as this drug can cause hair loss and an increased appetite (resulting in weight gain). If this is what is worrying your daughter, then talking to someone outside the family such as a specialist epilepsy nurse (if there is one in your area) or anyone else whom she respects and feels able to trust may help a lot.

Whatever we suggest, at the end of the day it is up to young people with epilepsy themselves whether or not they continue taking medication for their seizures. Parents and medical personnel can only do their best to provide accurate advice and information in a sensitive way which will hopefully enable these young people to make sensible and informed choices.

SURGERY

Can surgery be used to treat epilepsy?

It is becoming clear that surgery may actually cure epilepsy. A cure means that after surgery all anti-epileptic drugs can gradually be withdrawn and the person never has any more seizures. However, it is very important to understand that only a small percentage – perhaps no more than 4%–5% – of all people with epilepsy (ie children AND adults) have epilepsies which would be suitable for surgery and should actually be considered for it.

Are any special tests needed before surgery can be carried out?

Yes, children who may be suitable for surgical treatment will need special tests or investigations to try and find out from exactly where within the brain the epilepsy may be starting. These investigations cannot be done in any hospital: they must be carried out in a special epilepsy centre where the actual surgical operations are also performed.

The tests will include such things as brain scans (there is a section on *Scans* in Chapter 2) and videotelemetry, which has proved very useful in pre-surgical evaluation (it is described in the section on *EEGs*, also in Chapter 2). It will also be important to find out where the areas or 'centres' for speech and memory are located in the child's brain, to try to ensure that any operation will not cause any problems. This is particularly necessary for any operation that might be carried out in the temporal lobe (its location in the brain is shown in Figure 2 in Chapter 1).

How soon after diagnosis should epilepsy surgery be considered?

This is a difficult question to answer, but surgery should certainly be considered in the following situations:

- if the seizures are always partial or focal (ie beginning on one side of the body), occur frequently and do not come under control with two or, at most, three different anti-epileptic drugs;
- if the EEG and, more importantly, a brain scan (either a CT scan or, preferably, an MRI scan) shows a single abnormality in just one region of the brain (CT and MRI scans are discussed in the section on *Scans* in Chapter 2).

There are other times when surgery should perhaps be considered, but this will depend on the individual child and type of seizure or epilepsy.

It is also becoming clear that if surgery is to be undertaken it should be done sooner rather than later. In the past it was often delayed for many years as it was regarded as a 'treatment of last resort', but today doctors realise that if surgery is necessary and indicated, then the earlier it is performed, the better the outcome. This applies not only to the outcome for the epilepsy but also to the child's schooling and relationships with family and friends. It is therefore important to identify as soon as possible those children where the epilepsy is not going to respond to anti-epileptic drugs. The child's age does not matter, as there is no reason why surgery for epilepsy cannot be carried out in young infants. One of the youngest children ever operated on and reported in a scientific (medical) magazine was just a few months old. Children with learning difficulties may also be able to have epilepsy surgery.

Does epilepsy surgery always work?

There are many different types of operation which can be performed to try and cure or treat epilepsy, and they each have different success rates. The most successful operations are those which are carried out on the temporal lobe (its location in the brain is shown in Figure 2 in Chapter 1). Although most operations on the temporal lobe are performed in young adults, they are also carried out in children. Overall, up to 70% or 75% of people who have an operation for temporal lobe epilepsy will be 'cured' and will never have another seizure. Other types of operation do not have such high success rates, with only between 10% and 40% of people who have had such surgery being cured.

DIET

Do children with epilepsy need any special sort of diet?

No, not usually – but it is important for everyone to eat healthily, not just children who have epilepsy. This means choosing meals which are high in fibre, low in fat, and include plenty of fresh fruit and vegetables. It is important that meals are not missed, and strict weight-control diets are to be avoided. If you would like further information about what makes up a sensible diet, you could contact the Health

Education Authority (address in Appendix 2) which publishes booklets and leaflets on healthy eating.

A healthy body also needs rest and in some children disturbed sleep or long periods without sleep can trigger seizures. The occasional late night will not make any difference, but it is important to have a regular sleep pattern as part of a healthy lifestyle.

I have heard that it is possible to control seizures by eating a special sort of diet. Please could you tell me more about this?

Attempts have been made to control seizures by changing a child's diet. The best-known of these is called the 'ketogenic diet'. 'Ketogenic' comes from two other words: 'keto' from 'ketones', which are natural substances found in the blood and urine, and formed from the metabolism (breakdown in the body) of fats; and 'genic' meaning to produce or make. Thus the diet is literally one which 'makes lots of ketones'.

The ketogenic diet consists mainly of fat, is not very tasty, and therefore is usually not popular with either the child or the parents who have to make it up! It must be kept to very strictly and a hospital dietician will always need to be involved to ensure that it is worked out properly.

Doctors do not really know how the diet works in controlling seizures and, unfortunately, it does not always work. Even when it does, the effects may only last for a short time – only rarely do they last more than 12 months. Anti-epileptic drugs usually have to be continued along with the diet, although occasionally the drugs can be gradually reduced and even withdrawn. The ketogenic diet has a place in the treatment of a few children with difficult epilepsy, but it is not a suitable diet for the majority, and it is certainly not a 'cure-all' or alternative to anti-epileptic drugs.

COMPLEMENTARY THERAPIES

Do doctors disapprove of complementary or alternative medicines?

Before trying to answer this question, we need to make a distinction between medicines or therapies which claim to be 'alternatives' to treatments offered by the medical profession, and those which are 'complementary' and are meant to be used alongside conventional treatments. The use of a complementary therapy should be in addition to, not instead of, your child's usual anti-epileptic drugs. No one should stop taking their normal medication without a doctor's approval. This is particularly important with anti-epileptic drugs, where sudden withdrawal of treatment can be dangerous (this is discussed further in the sections on *Does treatment work?* and *Anti-epileptic drugs* earlier in this chapter).

The reservations held by many members of the medical and health professions largely revolve around the fact that very few of these treatments have been subjected to properly controlled research. This means that there is little hard evidence that the treatments really work. If and when they should be used in epilepsy, how effective they are and the precise ways they work have not been fully established.

Doctors may understandably get upset about alternative or complementary treatments when parents are tempted to stop their children's usual medication, when the therapies themselves have serious side-effects, and when they feel that parents are being misinformed and persuaded to spend large sums of money which they can ill afford. If these features are not present, most practising doctors will take a neutral or even an encouraging view of complementary therapies and appreciate that, even if the scientific evidence for them is elusive or even nonexistent, they may still do some good. Sometimes just the feeling that you are doing something which may help your child can be very valuable.

My teenage daughter is keen to try a complementary therapy, I think mainly because she has read so much about them in the magazines she buys in the newsagents. But there seems to be

**such a lot of them – how do we decide which to try, and how do
we find someone to consult?**

The answers to the remaining questions in this section will
give you some idea of the complementary therapies which
have been used by people with epilepsy. Whichever you
choose to try, the most important thing is to find a practitioner who is adequately qualified. At the moment there is
nothing to prevent someone with minimal training – or even
no training at all – setting themselves up in business as a
practitioner and treating clients. In untrained hands, complementary therapies can do harm. However, the reputable
members of the various complementary therapies are trying
hard to improve their own practices and to give the public
more information about their qualifications and training.

There are a number of organisations representing complementary therapy practitioners: usually each therapy has
its own 'governing body' and there are also umbrella
organisations trying to improve standards across the whole
range of complementary treatments. You will find the
relevant addresses listed in the *HEA Guide to Complementary Medicine and Therapies* (details in Appendix 3),
which also includes suggestions on how to find a suitable
practitioner and the questions you should ask before
agreeing to a course of treatment. You could also ask at
your own GP's surgery or health centre for the names of
reputable local practitioners. Some practices now offer
some complementary therapies themselves.

Cost may be another factor that you want to take into
consideration. These therapies are not often available on the
NHS, and they can prove expensive.

Whichever therapy you and your daughter choose, and
however you find a practitioner, there are some things
which you must remember. Your daughter should talk to
her doctor before starting on her chosen therapy, to make
quite sure that it will not interfere or interact in any way

with her medical treatment. She must tell the complementary practitioner about her epilepsy, and she must continue to take her anti-epileptic drugs as usual.

I saw a television programme which showed people altering their brainwaves by watching a computer screen. What were they doing, and is it useful in treating epilepsy?

This is a technique called biofeedback. It is based on the fact that it is easier to learn how to alter some aspect of your physical or mental state (ie to develop conscious control of your body's reactions) if you get some sort of reward each time you manage to make the desired change (the 'feedback' part of the name – 'bio' simply means life). Have you ever taught yourself to wink or to raise just one eyebrow or anything similar by looking in the mirror while you were trying to do it? If so, you were using a very simple form of biofeedback – seeing your success in the mirror made it easier for you to repeat the action another time.

The monitoring devices used in biofeedback are rather more sophisticated than mirrors – they can measure such things as muscle tension, heart rate, breathing pattern, blood pressure, perspiration and so on. When you succeed in achieving your aim (perhaps to relax a specific muscle, or stop your palms sweating) then the monitor gives you some sort of reward: you might move a pointer, or make a sound louder, or completely change a screen image (on the versions which use computers). The reward reinforces your ability to do the same thing again.

Research has begun into the use of biofeedback in epilepsy because some people have been able to learn to alter their brainwave patterns using this technique (brainwaves are explained in the section on *EEGs* in Chapter 2). Obviously if it could be shown that this was possible for everyone, then there might be a chance that at some time in the future people with epilepsy could learn to control their brainwaves and in turn perhaps control their seizures. However, the research is still in the very early stages and we cannot expect it to bear fruit for many years (if at all). Certainly the biofeedback therapies available from a complementary practitioner cannot be used to control epilepsy, although they can be helpful aids to relaxation.

What is aromatherapy? Is it true that it can be used to help people with epilepsy and, if so, can it be used on children?

Aromatherapy is a complementary therapy involving treatment with essential oils, which are aromatic (scented) oils extracted from the roots, flowers or leaves of plants by distillation. Aromatherapy often involves massage, but the oils can also be inhaled or added to baths.

Interest in aromatherapy has grown rapidly in the general population over recent years, so it is not surprising that some people with epilepsy have explored the possibility of using this therapy to help control their seizures. Some people with epilepsy use aromatherapy as a form of relaxation, as they believe that reducing stress in this way in turn reduces the frequency of their seizures. There are also people with epilepsy who experience an 'aura' before they have a seizure – a warning (usually involving a strange sensation, feeling, smell or taste) that a seizure is about to happen. A few of these people have found that smelling a particular aromatherapy oil (usually lavender, chamomile, ylang ylang or bergamot) as soon as they notice the aura can prevent the seizure happening.

Unfortunately all the evidence for the use of aromatherapy in epilepsy is anecdotal – there have been no properly controlled medical research trials of whether it actually works or not. We know of only one small and informal hospital study into its use, and that involved only a couple of dozen adults and no children. We need to wait for proper research to be set up and the results published before we can say for certain whether or not aromatherapy can definitely help in epilepsy (or not, as the case may be). We will not have an answer for a number of years.

In the meantime, we can certainly say that aromatherapy is a pleasant means of relaxation which can be used by children as well as adults, providing that all the precautions we have mentioned elsewhere in this section are followed (eg conventional treatment with anti-epileptic drugs must be continued). It is particularly important to find a properly qualified aromatherapist: people with epilepsy should avoid those practitioners whose qualifications are in the use of aromatherapy as a beauty treatment rather than as a complementary therapy. Aromatherapists would also recommend that you avoid buying the essential oils available over the counter in health food shops without taking proper advice first, as not only do they vary in quality, but some of them can actually increase seizure frequency (examples include rosemary, sweet fennel, camphor, hyssop and sage) and so should not be used.

What complementary therapies have been tried for epilepsy? Do any of them actually work?

At a guess, probably all of them by some people with epilepsy somewhere in the world! However, apart from those already mentioned earlier in this section, the ones which are most likely to be tried are the following.

- **Acupuncture**
  This is a traditional form of Chinese medicine which involves inserting special very fine needles into the skin at particular sites on the body in order to balance the 'life energy' or 'vital force' which the Chinese call 'ch'i' or 'qi'.

- **Homeopathy**
  This therapy is based on the principle that 'like can be cured with like' (the word homeopathy comes from two Greek words that mean 'similar' and 'suffering'). The

remedies used contain very dilute amounts of a substance which in larger quantities would produce similar symptoms to the illness being treated. Homeopathic doctors believe that illness is caused by imbalances within the body and they concentrate on strengthening the body's natural defences. Homeopathic remedies should only be used after a discussion with both a doctor and a qualified homeopathic specialist (homeopathy is available through the NHS although the provision is limited).

- **Hypnotherapy**
  A person who is hypnotised enters a state of very deep relaxation, during which they are more receptive to suggestions of ways of altering behaviour than they would be in a fully-conscious state. While it is most useful in reinforcing good intentions to change bad habits (eg stopping smoking), it can also be helpful in reducing stress and increasing confidence.

- **Relaxation**
  Some complementary therapies (eg massage) encourage relaxation, but it is also possible to learn how consciously to relax at will, either at classes or by listening to special cassette tapes.

The real use of all the complementary therapies we have described is in aiding relaxation and helping relieve some of the stress and anxiety which may be found in people with epilepsy, particularly teenagers and young adults. This suggests that sometimes they would seem to be more useful for the parents of a child with epilepsy, rather than for the children themselves! If you are considering one of these treatments for your child, then remember to take his or her wishes into account – being an unwilling participant will only increase stress and worry, not reduce them.

Some people will claim that these complementary therapies are useful in epilepsy, but it is extremely unlikely that any of these methods are effective by themselves: anti-epileptic drugs will still be needed. In other words, they really are complementary – they are a complement to, not an alternative to or substitute for, conventional treatment with anti-epileptic drugs. But as long as these different treatments do not interact or interfere with a child's conventional treatment, there is no reason why they should not be tried. As already mentioned, it is important to discuss all non-medical treatment with your doctor before embarking on any course of complementary therapy for your child's seizures.

CHAPTER 4

Is it an emergency?

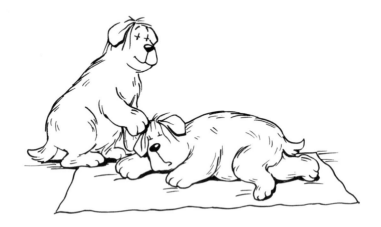

INTRODUCTION

Is a seizure an emergency? More often than not, the answer to this question is no. But everyone should know what to do when a seizure occurs (or what not to do, which is equally important), as well as how to recognise an emergency and what to do in those circumstances.

One situation which is definitely an emergency is status epilepticus. Although status epilepticus is rare, when it occurs it is potentially a very serious condition, and so it has its own section at the end of this chapter.

All the types of seizure mentioned in this chapter are explained in more detail in the sections on *Types of epilepsy* and *More about seizures* in Chapter 1.

FIRST AID

Can you give us some general first aid rules for what to do when a child has a seizure?

First aid is not required for most types of seizure (although there are exceptions, including generalised tonic-clonic seizures and complex partial seizures, and these are dealt with in the following questions in this section). All seizures should be allowed to run their natural course: recovery times will vary from child to child, and will also depend on the type of seizure. Try not to panic, and if the child is frightened by the seizure, then be reassuring.

Our daughter wanders in her seizures. What should we do?

Children who wander during a seizure usually have complex partial seizures, during which they may behave strangely and they may appear confused. General first aid advice is as follows:

- be understanding and talk gently and reassuringly to your daughter while the seizure is continuing;
- only attempt physical contact with her if she appears to be at risk of harming herself, in which case move her gently away from danger;
- if there is no danger, let the seizure take its natural course.

John has generalised tonic-clonic epilepsy. What can we do when he has one of his major convulsive seizures? What is safe?

Some general first aid advice for this type of seizure is as follows:

- help his breathing by turning him onto his side and, if possible, into the recovery position (shown in Figure 14), and loosening any tight clothing;
- protect him from injury by moving furniture or other hard objects out of his way;

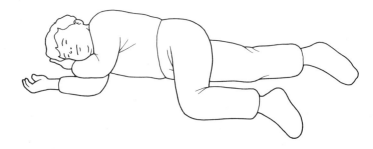

Figure 14: Recovery position.

- protect his head from injury, eg by putting a cushion, pillow or folded-up sweater or coat underneath it, or by using your hands or arms;
- do not move him unless he is in immediate danger, eg has fallen near a fire or on a staircase; and
- do not leave him alone until he is fully recovered.

One thing you very definitely should NOT do is to attempt to put anything between his teeth. This is not safe, and could cause considerable damage to his teeth. It could also result in you receiving an unpleasant bite.

When his lips go blue, is it dangerous? Do we need to call the doctor?

Blueness around the mouth (called perioral cyanosis) is caused by a low level of oxygen in the blood (it is discussed in more detail in the section on *More about seizures* in Chapter 1). It is usually self-limiting: a pink colour returns rapidly once the seizure has ended and normal oxygen levels have returned. It is not dangerous in itself, and medical help will only be needed if the seizure does not end spontaneously within a few minutes (when to call for help is discussed in the next section in this chapter).

Is it safe to let a child fall asleep after a seizure?

Yes. Most generalised tonic-clonic seizures are followed by

a period of sleep, which may last from half an hour up to several hours. This is normal following this type of seizure and is part of the post-ictal phase (ie what happens after a seizure). A child may also fall asleep after a complex partial seizure. Recovery times following seizures vary from child to child, but as long they are not left unattended and are kept under observation, it is safe to let them sleep for however long they need.

Should all parents learn how to give their children Stesolid as a first aid measure?

No. Parents only need to learn when and how to use Stesolid (rectal diazepam) if their child has epilepsy which is firstly difficult to control and secondly likely to lead to frequent and long seizures. If this is the case for your child, then you will be taught about Stesolid; if it is not, then you are unlikely ever to need it (you could check with your doctor about this if you are at all concerned). Stesolid is almost never needed for children with typical absence epilepsy or BREC (benign rolandic epilepsy of childhood). It is more likely to be required for children with severe myoclonic epilepsy or the Lennox-Gastaut syndrome.

Stesolid is the brand name for one formulation of one particular anti-epileptic drug whose generic name is diazepam. It is a solution which comes in a small tube with a nozzle which is inserted into a child's rectum (the back passage, also referred to as the anus). Clearly a drug cannot be given by mouth during a seizure as the child will be unable to swallow, but giving the drug into the rectum is effective because it is well absorbed into the blood stream from there.

CALLING AN AMBULANCE

Should I call my GP every time my daughter has a seizure?

In most cases the answer to this question is no, but there will be exceptions, and your daughter may be one of them. We would suggest that you talk it over with your GP and decide between you if and when you should call the surgery or health centre. There are circumstances when calling for emergency help is necessary (which will mean dialling 999 for an ambulance rather than ringing your GP) and these are listed in the answer to the next question.

At what stage during a seizure or a series of seizures should someone call an ambulance?

Emergency medical care should be considered in the following circumstances:

- if a second or third seizure occurs without the child regaining consciousness;
- if the convulsive part of the seizure is lasting longer than usual for your child, and certainly if it lasts longer than 10 minutes;
- if any injuries have occurred during the seizure, eg cuts requiring stitches;
- if the cause of the seizure is uncertain and further investigation is necessary; or
- if for any other reason you are worried or concerned about your child either during or after the seizure.

What happens to the child once the ambulance arrives?

First of all, it is important that whenever possible someone who saw the child's seizure (the eyewitness) gives a detailed account to the paramedics or the ambulance crew on their arrival. They will assess the situation and administer emergency first aid should that be necessary. Once in the ambulance, a member of the crew will remain with the child until they arrive at the Accident and Emergency Department of the hospital.

Should someone go to the hospital with the child?

Yes, if at all possible, for two reasons. The first is that children will obviously feel less scared and worried if they have a parent or someone else they know with them. Ask the ambulance crew if you can travel in the ambulance with your child but if for some reason this is not possible, then get to the hospital as soon as you can.

The second reason is that the person who saw the seizure (the eyewitness, who will not necessarily be one of the child's parents) will be needed at the hospital to tell the doctors in the Accident and Emergency Department exactly what happened. It is not essential for eyewitnesses to travel in the ambulance, but the doctors will want to talk to them as soon as possible after the child has reached the hospital, so they do need to get there quickly.

What happens when they reach the hospital?

On arrival at the hospital the child will be given a thorough medical examination by a doctor. A medical history will be taken, and it is important that a detailed account of the seizure is given to the hospital staff (the importance of eyewitness accounts is explained in the section *How do they know it's epilepsy?* in Chapter 2).

What happens next depends on whether or not the seizures have stopped. If the seizures are continuing, then emergency medical help will be required: the child may be given rectal diazepam (discussed in the previous section in this chapter) or intravenous anti-epileptic drugs or both. If, on the other hand, the seizure has stopped and the child is in a post-ictal condition (post-ictal means 'after the seizure'), then he or she may remain in the hospital for a period of observation. This may be for a few hours, or perhaps overnight, depending upon a number of factors including how well the child is, whether there is another medical condition which may have caused the seizure and which needs treating, and the wishes of the parents.

STATUS EPILEPTICUS

What is status epilepticus?

The currently internationally-accepted definition of status epilepticus (a Latin phrase which simply means 'in an epileptic condition') is either:

- any seizure lasting for at least 30 minutes; or
- repeated seizures lasting for 30 minutes or longer, from which the person did not regain consciousness between each seizure.

Any type of seizure may develop into status epilepticus, although few do – fortunately it is a rare condition. Generalised tonic-clonic seizures are the most likely to lead to status epilepticus: this is called convulsive status epilepticus, and is the most serious type. The other type is called non-convulsive status epilepticus and may occur in absence epilepsy and with complex partial seizures. It is easy for doctors to recognise convulsive status epilepticus, but non-convulsive absence status and particularly non-convulsive complex partial status may be more difficult to diagnose. EEGs are very important in diagnosing non-convulsive status epilepticus (there is a section on *EEGs* in Chapter 2).

Convulsive and non-convulsive status epilepticus are medical and neurological emergencies and need to be treated quickly. If you think that your child is in status epilepticus, then call for help immediately (as discussed in the previous section on *Calling an ambulance*).

Can status epilepticus be caused by propping a child up during a seizure?

This would be very unlikely. From a safety point of view, however, it would be unwise to prop a child up during a generalised tonic-clonic seizure. Wherever possible it is best to leave the child lying down on his or her side, as described in the *First aid* section at the beginning of this chapter.

Can status epilepticus cause brain damage?

Epilepsy rarely causes brain damage. Convulsive status epilepticus (explained earlier in this section) may cause brain damage, but only if it is not treated promptly. The only situation where recurrent generalised or partial seizures may cause brain damage are if either:

- the seizures are so frequent (ie happening every few minutes for days at a time) that the child (and the brain) does not recover between seizures; or
- a single seizure (usually a tonic-clonic seizure or convulsion) lasts for more than 60 or 90 minutes without stopping.

Is status epilepticus life threatening?

It can be, but the risks today are far less than they used to be. Fewer than 3% of children with status epilepticus die these days, compared to approximately 10% in 1970. This is because firstly convulsive status epilepticus is not as common as it used to be, and secondly because it is diagnosed and treated more rapidly.

However, today's lower risks do not make status epilepticus any less serious. Convulsive and non-convulsive status epilepticus (both defined earlier in this section) are medical and neurological emergencies, and the outcome depends on the time interval between the seizures beginning and the start of effective treatment. Convulsive status epilepticus may be life threatening, particularly if it lasts 60 minutes or longer (which is very rare). Non-convulsive status is not life threatening, but it is still a medical emergency as it can sometimes change into convulsive status.

CHAPTER 5

Feelings, families and friends

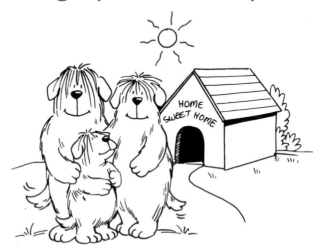

INTRODUCTION

Being told that your child has epilepsy is bound to be a shock, and many thoughts and feelings will flash through your mind. Different people will react in different ways: some will feel worried and depressed, others angry or guilty. Some parents will find the diagnosis a relief as they have been imagining something much worse, others will want to blot out the news completely in the hope it will just go away. These are all very natural reactions, as are your worries about how your family and friends will respond when you tell them about it.

COMING TO TERMS WITH EPILEPSY

Are conditions such as epilepsy really discussed more openly these days? Our GP seems to be suggesting that it would be a

good idea for us to talk to each other more about our daughter's epilepsy, or perhaps even to talk to other parents in our position, but we really don't know where to start.

We think they are talked about more openly these days (although we can't prove it). Epilepsy and other medical conditions are certainly discussed more openly on television and radio and in the press than was the case a few years ago.

When it comes to talking on a more personal level, then everyone is different. Some people will find it easy to talk about, but for many families this is not the case. There are any number of reasons for this reluctance, ranging from not wanting to accept the diagnosis to simple embarrassment at discussing personal feelings. Of course it takes time to adjust to being told that your child has epilepsy but in our experience being able to talk about it can help, even when sharing your feelings is difficult.

Finding out more about epilepsy from as many sources as possible is a good way to increase your family's confidence in discussing it. As epilepsy is a very common condition in children, you will soon discover that many other families have been in your situation. Your own particular experiences will of course be unique to you and your family, but you will find that many of them will be similar to those of others. The various epilepsy associations are good starting places for finding out more about epilepsy, and you will find their addresses in Appendix 1.

If you feel it would be helpful to talk to someone outside your family, then you could ask your doctor or your local epilepsy group to put you in touch with other families where there is a child with epilepsy, or perhaps with an experienced counsellor. If there is an epilepsy specialist nurse in your area then she would be another source of help, information and support.

I am feeling so guilty. Could we have done anything to prevent our child developing epilepsy?

Feeling guilty is common, not just among parents of children with epilepsy, but also among parents of children with diabetes, cerebral palsy or any one of a host of other conditions. There is rarely anything anyone could have done to change things. Epilepsy in most children just appears without a reason and is no one's fault. It is understandable that you may feel this way and it may take time for you to convince yourself otherwise, but there really is no reason why you should blame yourself. You might find it helpful to talk to other parents in the same position as yourself, and we suggested ways of making contact with them in the answer to the previous question.

My husband is very upset about our daughter and won't help at all, he seems to just want to ignore it. What can I do?

Everyone in a family needs time to come to terms with epilepsy, and often the last person to accept the diagnosis is the father. The reasons why can be many, but you and your daughter will need his help and support, both now and in the future. It is in everyone's interests that all members of the family are pulling in the same direction. Fathers sometimes choose to opt out, but in other cases they can be inadvertently left out, especially if pressure of work or family circumstances prevent them spending much time with their children.

Try to encourage him to talk about his feelings as soon as possible, if not to you then to a friend, your doctor or an epilepsy specialist nurse (if you have one in your area). Talking to him about your own feelings and how much you value his support might be a possible starting point. If he is reluctant to discuss things, then perhaps you could persuade him to go to the GP's or the hospital with you for your daughter's next appointment, to encourage him to feel involved.

Epilepsy scares me. Will this fear ever go away?

Being told that your child has epilepsy can be frightening, especially if you know little about it. Learning more about epilepsy can help, as can talking about your fears and worries (we have suggested ways of finding someone to talk to in earlier answers in this section).

Above all you need to give yourself time to come to terms with the diagnosis. It is a bit like a bereavement – you have lost something (your child's complete good health) and you need to give yourself the opportunity to grieve for your loss and accept it. The fear will gradually subside as you gain experience and confidence. You may never lose it completely, but it will no longer be at the forefront of your mind all the time.

How much should we tell our son about his epilepsy?

We would recommend that you tell him as much as possible (so long as he is willing to listen!) but without being over-dramatic or placing an overemphasis on the place of his epilepsy in his life.

Epilepsy is often difficult to explain in an understandable form to a young child, but there is now some help available in the form of excellent written materials and videos designed for younger children who have epilepsy but who are otherwise healthy. Unfortunately materials for children who have learning difficulties in addition to epilepsy are virtually non-existent. When it comes to older children you have a choice. Depending on their abilities, you could use some of the materials designed for adults, but if you feel that would not be appropriate then there are some materials available specifically aimed at adolescents. The best way forward is to contact the epilepsy associations (addresses in Appendix 1) and ask for their literature and video lists.

If your son is willing to learn about and discuss his epilepsy, then please make it as easy as possible for him to do so. The sooner he feels in control of his condition the easier his life will be. Some children as young as 7 and 8 are able to take control of their medication and other aspects of their own management, but this can only be achieved by giving them information in an understandable form in the first place.

Since our daughter's diagnosis, we have always made sure that she is never alone, especially when she goes out. Either her father or I always stay with her. She is now becoming very rebellious, and is refusing to go to play at her friends' houses unless she is allowed to do so on her own. We don't see how she can be safe unless one of us is there, so how can we persuade her that we are staying with her for her own good?

Without knowing more about your daughter (how old she is, the nature of her epilepsy and how long it has been since her diagnosis) we can only give a very general answer. All parents worry about their children learning to cope with the world, and parents of children with epilepsy probably worry more than most. The temptation is to wrap them in cotton wool and try to protect them from any possible harm.

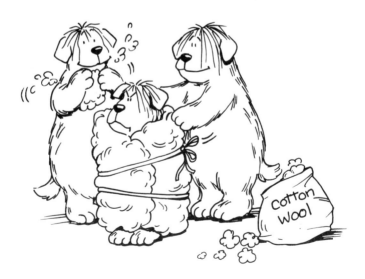

Colour Section

LIST OF PLATES

Plate 1 DRUG AND TRADEMARK TABLES

All drugs have at least two names. The generic name is the basic drug name, but each drug also has a brand name, given by the manufacturer. The generic and brand names of the most commonly used anti-epileptic drugs are given in Table A.

The brand names of the drugs are registered trademarks, belonging to particular manufacturers, and these are listed in Table B.

A selection of these drugs are illustrated as colour plates for your information.

Table A: Generic and brand names of drugs

Generic name	Brand names
acetazolamide	Diamox
carbamazepine	Tegretol, Tegretol Retard
clobazam	Frisium
clonazepam	Rivotril
ethosuximide	Emeside, Zarontin
gabapentin	Neurontin
lamotrigine	Lamictal
phenytoin	Epanutin
primidone	Mysoline
sodium valproate	Epilim, Epilim Chrono
topiramate	Topamax
valproic acid	Convulex
vigabatrin	Sabril

Table B: Trademarks

Brand name	Manufacturer
Convulex	Pharmacia
Diamox	Storz
Epilim, Epilim Chrono	Sanofi Winthrop
Emeside	L.A.B.
Epanutin	Parke-Davis
Frisium	Hoechst Marion Roussel
Lamictal	Glaxo Wellcome
Mysoline	Zeneca
Neurontin	Parke-Davis
Rivotril	Roche
Sabril	Hoechst Marion Roussel
Tegretol, Tegretol Retard	CIBA
Topamax	Janssen-Cilag
Zarontin	Parke-Davis

Plate 2   LAMICTAL

Lamictal (generic name lamotrigine) is available in a range of different strength tablets or dispersible tablets. Remember, always discuss your medication with your doctor or nurse. Packaging and tablets not to scale.

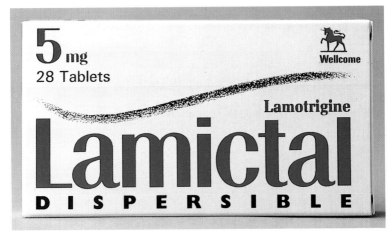

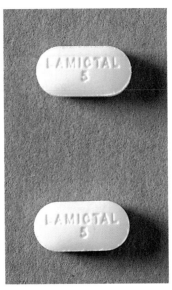

Plate 3   SABRIL

Sabril (generic name vigabatrin) is available in tablet or sachet form. Remember, always discuss your medication with your doctor or nurse. Packaging and tablets not to scale.

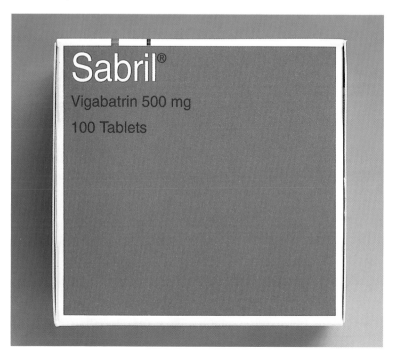

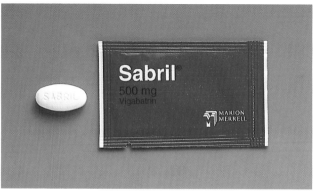

Plate 4   NEURONTIN

Neurontin (generic name gabapentin) is available as capsules only, in a range of different strengths. It is currently not licensed for use with children under 12. Remember, always discuss your medication with your doctor or nurse. Packaging and tablets not to scale.

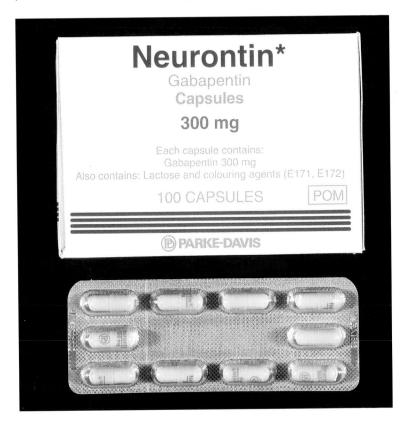

Plate 5   TOPAMAX

Topamax (generic name topiramate) is available in a range of different strength tablets. It is currently not licensed for use with children. Remember, always discuss your medication with your doctor or nurse. Packaging and tablets not to scale.

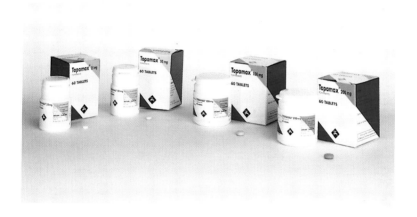

Plate 6   TEGRETOL

Tegretol (generic name carbamazepine) is available as a liquid, conventional tablets, controlled release tablets, chewable tablets or as suppositories (for short term use only). The illustration shows Tegretol Retard 200 mg tablets, which are designed to be taken twice a day. Remember, always discuss your medication with your doctor or nurse. Packaging and tablets not to scale.

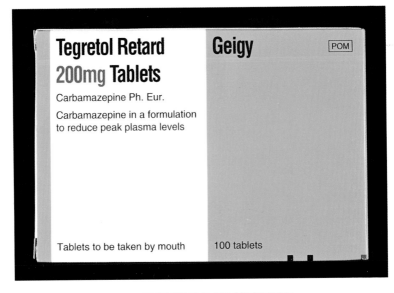

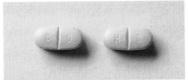

However, children with epilepsy have the same needs as other children. If they are to grow up and develop into independent adults, then they have to learn to do things by themselves and take the everyday risks of life without unnecessary restrictions. We all take risks every day (think how often you cross the road!) and it is only through experience that we know how to calculate what we can and cannot do with reasonable safety.

It sounds from your question as if your daughter is old enough to start taking responsibility for herself, and we would suggest that you encourage her to do so. Perhaps you could start slowly: you could take her to and collect her from her friends' homes but leave her there to play, having made sure that anyone with her knows what to do if she has a seizure and where to contact you in an emergency. Then, as your confidence increases, you could allow her to do more and more on her own. We are not suggesting that you should throw all caution to the winds, simply that you try to balance the need for sensible precautions with your daughter's understandable desire to be treated like other children.

Our 12-year-old son will now only leave the house to go to school – he refuses to go out with his friends or to come on family outings, he won't even go to the shops to spend his pocket money. Could this be because of his drugs (although he's been on the same one for several years now)?

They could be the reason, although it sounds unlikely if his treatment has not changed recently. It would certainly be worth checking with his doctor to see if it might be the case.

However, there are other and perhaps more likely possibilities. The first is his age – he could simply be displaying typical grumpy adolescent behaviour. His refusal even to go to the shops on his own makes it sound rather more than that, so perhaps he is worried about his epilepsy.

Has anything happened recently to make him lose his

confidence? Perhaps he had a seizure at school and he has been told exaggerated stories about how he looked, or someone may be teasing or bullying him because of his epilepsy. Can you persuade him to talk about what is worrying him? If you can, then you will be able to provide some reassurance while at the same time acknowledging his fears. Once the problem is out in the open, then you can start to restore his confidence. If teasing is the cause, then you can deal with it (this is discussed in the section on *Getting on at school* in Chapter 6); if he has been told silly stories about his behaviour during a seizure, then you can give him the true facts; if he is worried about being out on his own, then you could arrange for someone to be with him until he begins to feel more self-reliant and decides that he no longer needs your support.

Do you think a person with epilepsy should be described as that, or as an 'epileptic'? I dislike it when I hear someone refer to my daughter as an 'epileptic', but I don't want to make any unnecessary fuss about it.

Your daughter now has a diagnosis of epilepsy, but is this a reason to use any labels? Depending on how you and others treat her, she will be the same person she was before and giving her any sort of label will not help. Your daughter and her epilepsy will both be very individual and should be treated as such, not labelled.

As you will have gathered, in our opinion labels like 'epileptic' are very unhelpful although unfortunately they are still used frequently, especially by some professionals who should know better. However, informing people calmly and politely of your feelings about this can hardly be considered to be making a fuss.

FAMILY FEELINGS

Our youngest child has been diagnosed with epilepsy, and now

our eldest daughter is terrified she will develop it as well. What should we do?

Your daughter is understandably upset by the diagnosis of epilepsy in your youngest child, and her fear is a very common response. You can reassure her that there is no reason why her own health status should change, as the chances of her developing epilepsy herself are very small. Encourage her to keep everything in perspective: learning more about epilepsy may help with this, as knowing the facts will enable her to cope with her fears.

Sandra's brother hates her epilepsy, because he says his friends no longer want to come to our house to play. How can we help him overcome this?

Your son's friends may be frightened because they do not understand what epilepsy is, and he may be reinforcing this by expressing negative views about it to them (he may still feel frightened himself). Reassurance should help – perhaps you could explain to them what epilepsy is and how little they would have to do if Sandra has a seizure while they are playing at your house (basic epilepsy first aid is described in Chapter 4). Your son's self-confidence could be lower than usual and this will take time to recover, so some positive conversations about epilepsy are probably required. When your son feels reassured, then you could encourage him to talk positively about Sandra's epilepsy to his friends.

We cannot leave Anne alone with her 18-year-old brother, because he says he cannot cope with her seizures. What can we do?

First aid for seizures is usually easy and you need to help your son appreciate this. Good first aid information is freely available from the various epilepsy associations (addresses in Appendix 1) and you could encourage him to read this or similar information from other sources (the section on *First aid* in Chapter 4, for example). You could also try to involve him in managing a seizure whilst you are there as this should help to build up his confidence to deal with any that happen when he is alone with Anne.

These suggestions should help on a practical level, but only you can know how good your son is at expressing his feelings. It may be that he has other worries that he finds it more difficult to talk about: for example, he may be feeling left out of the family because he thinks everyone is concentrating on Anne, or he may be being teased by his friends because he is expected to take care of his sister. If you think that this may be the case, then you will need to encourage him to talk about his real concerns so that you can work out how to deal with them.

My parents will no longer allow my son to sleep at their house at weekends. This is distressing all of us, especially my son who loves staying with his grandparents. I don't know what to say to convince them that it would be all right, can you suggest anything?

Grandparents often find it very hard to accept epilepsy in their family. When they were younger epilepsy was usually discussed in a very negative way (if it was discussed at all), and because of this they may have inaccurate ideas about it. Taking charge of other people's children is always a major responsibility, and they may be frightened of any harm coming to your son while he is staying with them.

As with so many other similar situations, the answer here is communication. Can you encourage your parents to learn more about epilepsy and to talk about their worries? Perhaps they could come with you and your son when you go to the hospital to see the specialist. If you have an epilepsy specialist nurse in your area, then you might be able to arrange for her to visit your parents to talk about epilepsy in more detail and discuss their concerns with them.

If you have room at home, perhaps your parents could come to stay with you for a few weekends. This could give you the opportunity to explain what needs to be done, if anything, if your son has a seizure. Reassure them that it is simple and then hopefully with a little persuasion and confidence-building they will let him stay with them once more. Perhaps you could go with him the first few times until they feel less apprehensive?

OUTSIDE THE FAMILY

My husband and I are trying to work out how to tell other people about our child's diagnosis. At the moment we can't even decide who needs to know. Can you help us make up our minds?

Almost everyone will have to share news about health issues at some time in their lives, and news about epilepsy is no different. If you are worried about people's reactions, then you will probably be pleasantly surprised. Ask the people you tell what they would like to know: each response will be different, but they are more likely to be interested and concerned rather than discomforted. If you do come across a negative reaction, it will probably be caused by ignorance, and you should be able to overcome it by providing information about epilepsy and talking about it in a positive way.

One reason why you need to tell your family and friends is that you will probably need their help if you are to carry on with your life as before – perhaps you will want them to babysit for you, or to take your child out for the day with their children, and so on. If you were worried about your child's health before diagnosis, then they will probably be aware of this, so the sooner they know the truth the better (if you do not tell them, they may be imagining problems far worse than epilepsy).

When it comes to people that you know less well, then only you can decide what is appropriate. You must tell people who will have to take responsibility for your child such as the teachers at school, Scout or Guide leaders, and so on (you will find more information about this in other chapters of this book, eg Chapter 6 on *School* and Chapter 9 on *Your Child's Social Life*). You may want to tell your neighbours, even if they are only acquaintances rather than friends, and you may also want to tell someone at work, in case you need to arrange time off for hospital appointments. Whatever you decide, take a positive approach in the telling: being positive yourself invites a positive reaction.

Since we told our friends about our daughter's epilepsy, there is one couple that we hardly seem to see any more, we think because they are frightened of it. We want to carry on as normal, so what can we do? Can we really still expect them to make us welcome?

People can be apprehensive about epilepsy for many different reasons, so you will need to try and find out what is really bothering your friends and then provide them with the information that will help to reassure them. After your conversation, give them some time to absorb what you have told them and adjust to it, and then we would hope that they would be as welcoming as before. You might discover that your worries about them were unfounded, and that they thought they were behaving in a helpful way. Perhaps they wanted you to have time to adjust to the diagnosis without being worried by social calls, or they may have simply not known how to talk to you about it.

All the people who know about our child's epilepsy have been very sympathetic, but we feel that they don't really understand that we just want to lead an ordinary life. This applies not just to our friends, but also to some of the medical staff that we meet. How can we make them understand what we want?

In other words, you don't want sympathy but you do want empathy. Some people will treat you sympathetically thinking that this is helpful, and you will need to try to explain to them just what it is that you want. Tell them that your family intends to live life as before and that constructive help to do this would be more than welcome. Only you can know what you consider to be constructive help – it may be something practical like collecting your child from school one day, or you may want someone to talk to about your feelings, or you may simply want them to stop asking you about your child's health every time you meet!

You may also have to discuss this issue with the medical staff. Some professionals will still provide you with a list of things your child should not do now that epilepsy has been diagnosed. This is a negative attitude, and it would be more useful for you to find out the facts about why children can still carry on with their usual activities rather than why they cannot.

CHAPTER 6

School

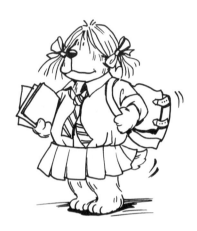

INTRODUCTION

As school is so important in children's lives, it is not surprising that parents have many specific questions to ask about it. However, teachers are not the only people who take responsibility for children in the absence of their parents, so many of our answers are equally applicable outside school. Anyone caring for your child will need to know something about epilepsy, and in most cases the information they need will be very similar to that outlined here.

TEACHING THE TEACHERS

Does the school need to know? Wouldn't it be easier if we kept the news to ourselves?

If you want your child to have a safe and active life then yes, the school does need to know. If you find it difficult to talk about your child's epilepsy then it might be easier for you not to mention it, but it would certainly not be better – the teachers' ignorance could lead to your child being inadvertently put at risk.

Most parents worry about a school's reaction to a diagnosis of epilepsy. We cannot predict what response you will get, but it will probably depend how much the staff already know about epilepsy. Some schools will be knowledgeable and very helpful, others may be less so. If you can take a positive attitude when you break the news, then you are more likely to get a positive response. We discuss whom and what to tell in the answers to the next few questions.

Generally speaking, the more information and knowledge teachers and schools have, the more understanding they will be – and this will help not just your child, but all children.

We realise that we must tell John's school, but we're not sure where to start. Who would be the best person to contact?

Different schools will have different policies about this, which will probably depend at least partly on the size of the school. Your first point of contact is most likely to be the head teacher, but in a larger school it might be a form (class) or year teacher, or a teacher with special responsibility for the children's welfare. If you were given some literature about John's school when he started there, then this might tell you who the correct person is, or you could telephone and ask the school secretary for this information. Another approach could be to start by telling a teacher that you already know quite well, and take their advice on what to do next.

Wherever you start, it is very important to emphasise that all the staff who come into contact with your son should be aware of his epilepsy, and this includes all the school meals and administrative staff as well as the teachers. They should either know what to do if a seizure occurs or whom to call for help. The more staff informed, the better.

Exactly what should we tell the school?

Do you mean about epilepsy in general or your child's epilepsy in particular? What you have to tell them about epilepsy in general will depend on how much they already know: you may find them very knowledgeable, or you may have to start with the basics (see the answer to the next question).

When it comes to your own child's epilepsy, then you will need to tell them:

- what your child's seizures look like;
- if your child gets any warning (aura) of a seizure;
- how long the seizures last;
- how long a rest your child needs after a seizure;
- what first aid may be required;

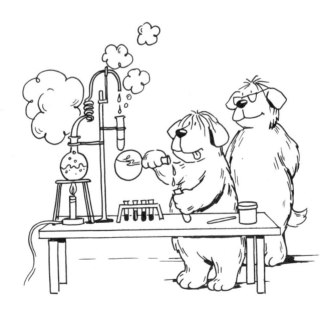

- how many seizures your child is having each week or month;
- if there is a pattern to the seizures or if you know of anything which makes them more likely to happen;
- if your child has to take any tablets or other forms of medication during the day and, if so, when they should be taken (you will probably also need to discuss their policy on medication brought into the school);
- if there are any side-effects from your child's drug treatment and, if so, what they are; and
- what action you would like the school to take if there is an emergency.

You will also want to discuss your child's lessons and other school activities, and explain what restrictions (if any) you think may be necessary. We would hope that in most cases these would be few, but you might want to ask for extra supervision during swimming or practical science or engineering lessons.

Our daughter's school is trying to be very helpful about her epilepsy, but it is very obvious that they actually know little about it. As her diagnosis is still very recent, we are still learning about it ourselves, and we find that we can't always answer their questions! Where can we get some help?

The various epilepsy associations produce special information packs for schools, and any of these would make a good starting point. Contact them at the addresses given in Appendix 1 for further details. You could also arrange for someone – perhaps an epilepsy specialist nurse or someone from a local epilepsy group – to come to the school to explain about epilepsy and answer questions. If you cannot find a suitable speaker yourself, then one of the associations may be able to suggest someone in your area.

Should the school look after Tracey's drugs for her, or can she just keep them with her?

As we know nothing about Tracey (not even her age), we can only answer your question in general terms. Our suggestions would obviously be different, for example, for a sensible teenager who is used to taking responsibility for her own drugs at home than for, say, a child who has learning difficulties as well as epilepsy and whose medication is always closely supervised (in which case all drugs should remain the responsibility of a teacher or a school nurse if there is one).

The first thing you will need to do is to find out her school's policy on prescription drugs, as these can vary considerably. Some schools have blanket procedures to cover all types of medication and all children, while others are more flexible and take the nature of the treatment and the child's age into account. Practical considerations are also important – Tracey should not simply carry her drugs around with her, so is there somewhere for her to keep them safely and out of reach of other children?

Teachers act 'in loco parentis' (a Latin phrase literally meaning 'in place of a parent'). This means that a teacher must take the same care of a child within his or her jurisdiction as would the child's own parents. This obviously places a considerable responsibility on school staff, and may lead them to appear over-cautious at times. At some schools teachers are reluctant to give prescription drugs to children, even when they need them – this means that a child's parents will often have to come in to school to give the medication.

Other schools insist that all drugs are kept by a member of staff. If this is the case, then Tracey should know where they are kept, at what time she has to take them, and what to do if the usual teacher in charge is away. Older children who are used to taking responsibility for their own treatment at home can resent having it supervised at school, and may react by 'forgetting' that they need a midday dose. If this happens and the school cannot alter its policy, then you could ask your GP or specialist if it would be possible to adjust Tracey's treatment so that she only needs to take her drugs once or twice a day instead of three or more times. Alternatively it might be possible for her (with her doctor's agreement) to take her so-called midday dose as soon as she returns home after school. Such adjustments could also be useful for a child who gets teased about taking treatment at school, or if a school is reluctant to provide suitable supervision.

Fortunately this whole issue of drugs in school is becoming less of a problem for children with epilepsy, because most of the modern anti-epileptic drugs only need to be given twice a day, which avoids the need for a dose during school hours.

Our son is sports-mad but his physical education teacher is reluctant to let him take part. Should we keep quiet and allow this?

No. Well-meaning people (not just teachers) can be over-protective of children, and even more so when a child has epilepsy. If you want your son to lead a full life then you will need to work out a way of dealing with this.

There are three factors you need to consider for any of your child's activities, whether at school or at home. These are the nature of the activity, your child's epilepsy, and what supervision is available. Consider the potential dangers of the activity, then decide whether your child's epilepsy would increase these potential dangers and, if so, what level of supervision would decrease them to a sensible level. If you do this, you are taking a logical approach to the problem.

You should discuss this logical approach with your son's physical education teacher and between you decide which activities will be possible. For example, you might decide it is not sensible for your son to work at heights in gymnastics, but that he could still take part in work at floor level. You might find out that the swimming pool can provide a member of staff to watch your son while he is swimming, which would mean he would be able to take part.

If you take each activity in isolation in this way then it will usually be possible to solve most problems. It may also be worth remembering that the child sitting at the side watching is sometimes more likely to have a seizure than the child taking part.

You can obviously apply this approach to other situations and activities, not just to sports. You could also use it with your son if you need to convince him that there is something he should not do without proper supervision!

There is a section on *Sports* in Chapter 9.

Our child is only 4 years old. Will his epilepsy stop him going to nursery school?

Everything we say about schools in this chapter can be applied equally well to nursery schools and playgroups. Providing you tell the staff about your son's epilepsy then there is no reason why he should not be able to attend and play an active part.

GETTING ON AT SCHOOL

Our daughter is being teased in school about her epilepsy. What can we do?

Fortunately this does not happen to all children, but unfortunately it does happen to some. Different children will have different reactions to being teased, so talk it over with your daughter and ask her if she would prefer to try to deal with this problem herself or whether she would like you to intervene. If she wants your help, then you could start by contacting her form teacher to see if between you you can make some progress.

If the teasing continues, it might be a good idea to see if the facts about epilepsy could be covered as part of the school's health education programme, emphasising that it is something that can happen to any child. This emphasis can often have the desired effect. The epilepsy associations will be able to provide suitable teaching materials if you contact them at the addresses given in Appendix 1.

We are worried about our child's current progress in school. Why may he be underachieving?

There are various reasons why this may be happening, not all of them connected with epilepsy. It is very easy for teachers and parents to blame epilepsy for a child's poor progress, but you do need to be very careful about doing this as it may mean that you are ignoring other causes.

If you are sure that his epilepsy is the cause, then the following are the most likely explanations you need to consider.

- A dislike of school because of teasing or difficulty in keeping up with other children.
- Teachers (and you?) assuming that your child will not achieve because of his epilepsy.
- Frequent seizures of any type, but especially absence seizures which are often not recognised, or – rarely – because of very frequent abnormal electrical activity in the brain which can only be detected by carrying out an EEG (there is a section on *EEGs* in Chapter 2).
- Damage to the brain, however minimal, which may affect just one aspect of learning (eg reading).
- Side-effects of anti-epileptic drugs (although this is not usually the most common cause) – most commonly drowsiness, poor memory, poor concentration.

You need to discuss all these factors with your son's teachers in an attempt to find out which appears to be the most important. You may find that more than one is a problem. Hopefully you will be able to solve any problems easily, but for some you may need the help of your doctor or another professional.

At a recent parents evening at Emma's school, her science teacher told us that she has been missing several of the lessons. Apparently Emma complains that she is 'feeling funny' so the teacher lets her go and lie down, worrying that making her attend the class will bring on a seizure. Can science lessons cause seizures?

No more than any other lessons! It sounds very much as if Emma is using her epilepsy as a way of avoiding a lesson she dislikes. Children are very skilled at using whatever they have to hand to manipulate adults in order to get out of something that they do not want to do (for example, homework makes a very good excuse for not cleaning your room or doing the washing up). Children with epilepsy are no different from others in this respect, they simply have a more believable excuse readily available. You will need to talk this through with Emma to find out if this is what she is doing.

However, there may be other reasons. Someone in her science class may be teasing her (teasing and how to deal with it is discussed in an earlier question in this section). She may have difficulties with the subject and find it stressful, and be genuinely worried that the stress will cause a seizure. If this is the case, you will need to help her learn ways of dealing with it. Stress is an inevitable part of life, and she will be happier in the long term if she learns how to cope with it rather than trying (and failing) to avoid it.

Our son is taking his GCSE exams this year. What happens if he has a seizure when he is taking an examination – how will it affect his results?

There are no definite rules, and policy does vary between

the examination boards, so the advice we can give here must be very general. Depending on how far he is through the examination and whether he is capable of continuing after the seizure, then the examination board may be willing to take into account the fact that he did have a seizure during the examination. His teacher will need to appeal to the board on his behalf outlining the exact facts, and this would certainly be worth doing should it unfortunately prove necessary. It will be easier for the board to come to a decision if the course concerned also has a major continuous assessment section.

Have you considered asking his school to contact the relevant board well in advance of his GCSEs to find out exactly what their attitude would be? It may also be helpful to have a letter from your son's doctor explaining his situation, particularly if his seizures are not well controlled.

Our son has fitted in well at junior school, but due to his quite severe epilepsy and slow progress academically should we consider a special school when he reaches 11?

This is an issue many parents of children with severe epilepsy have to face. It has been our experience that most junior schools cope with the integration of children with special needs more easily than secondary schools.

To find out what will be best in your case, you will need to discuss your worries and opinions with your son, with the schools concerned (his current school and the schools which he might attend at 11), and possibly with an educational psychologist from your local education authority. Your son may already have a statement of special educational needs (discussed in the answer to the next question) but if he does not, then this is a good time to ask his junior school about one. In theory this should lead to a thorough assessment of your son's abilities and should outline what extra help he might need during his future education. It sometimes leads to a recommendation for a special school placement or it may recommend providing extra support to allow him to attend a mainstream secondary school. The process of obtaining a statement can take a long time, so the earlier you ask about it the better.

I've heard about 'statements' before, but it's a piece of jargon that I don't understand. Please could you explain?

The 1981 Education Act was the start of statements of special educational needs. The Act stated that all children should, wherever possible, be integrated into mainstream schools. To make this possible, where necessary a 'statement' should be prepared of the educational needs of the child and the extra support that needed to be provided in the school. There have been other Education Acts since 1981 (eg the 1993 Education Act which laid down a code of practice for identifying and assessing children with special educational needs) but this system still stands.

We would advise any parent of a child with special needs to find out as much as possible about it from their local education authority, and to use it to get the best for their child (although this may take some persistence). The age of your child does not matter, as you do not have to wait until your child is old enough to go to school before starting the statementing process. The Department for Education and Employment publishes a booklet called *Special Educational Needs – A Guide for Parents* which outlines the procedures and explains the jargon used: details of how to obtain a copy are in Appendix 3.

CHAPTER 7

Practical concerns

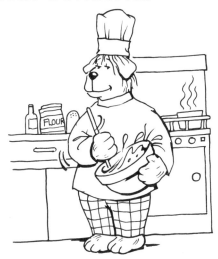

INTRODUCTION

This chapter is intended to answer many of the questions
that affect daily living when you have a child with epilepsy.
It covers a broad sweep of topics, from baths to benefits and
from doors to dentists. The common link is that they are all
'how to' concerns with practical answers.

SAFETY IN THE HOME

**My partner and I keep arguing about how many changes we
need to make in our home now that we have been told that our
daughter has epilepsy. I know things have to be safe, but I still
want her to grow up in a nice, normal home. Is this possible?**

Yes, of course. Without knowing more about your daughter
and her epilepsy we can only speak generally, but in most
cases the precautions you will need to take will only be

135

those you would make to keep any child safe. They should not have to affect the comfort of your home or be obvious to anyone else. For example, most parents will fit cooker and fire guards to prevent a child being accidentally burned – it makes no difference whether or not the child has epilepsy. You might need to rehang bathroom and lavatory doors so that they open outwards (then the door will not be blocked if your daughter falls behind it) but who will notice the difference?

It is a rare person who has never had an accident of some sort at home, and children (with or without epilepsy) are usually at more risk than adults. We should all probably take more care about home safety, particularly if we are parents. RoSPA (the Royal Society for the Prevention of Accidents – address in Appendix 2) produce information leaflets on the subject, which you might find useful. When you know that your home is reasonably safe for the whole family, then you can go on to consider any extra changes (if any) you may need to make to allow for your daughter's epilepsy. As you read the answers to the next few questions (which are about specific safety worries), remember that much of our advice would be equally applicable to every home, not just one in which there is a child with epilepsy.

Our daughter is very independent and often cooks for herself. Should we let her continue doing this now she has epilepsy?

In all but the most severe cases of epilepsy the answer is yes, but there are certain basic precautions she should take. A cooker guard would be sensible, and pan handles should always be turned inwards towards the cooker, not left sticking out into the room. She should also remember to take plates to pans rather than carrying saucepans containing boiling liquids. If you can afford one, a microwave oven would be safer than a conventional cooker.

What is the safest form of heating for our house now our young son has epilepsy?

All heating is potentially dangerous, but it is usually easy to protect children from the dangers whether or not they have epilepsy. Instead of spending a fortune on changing your heating system, why don't you just spend a little on fire or radiator guards? However, it would be best to avoid free-standing heaters.

Many of the inner doors in our house are mainly glass. Do we have to change them for solid doors?

Not necessarily. It might be safer in case your child has a seizure and falls into and breaks the glass panel, but if you like the doors you have then you could replace the original panels with safety glass. There are recommended standards for such glass and your local glass merchant should be able to advise you (you might discover that you already have safety glass fitted).

Our son has very frequent seizures involving falling and we are worried about the dangers our furniture presents. What can we do?

Some families in your situation have moved as much furniture as possible away from the middle of the room, especially in rooms where their child regularly plays or where the furniture is solid and has sharp edges. Some pad their furniture with soft materials like foam rubber, but others think that this alters the appearance of the home too much. It is quite easy to hide padding on chairs, tables and bed bases under covers or valances, more difficult to hide it on items such as cupboards and wardrobes. Other options are to move hard furniture to a room which your child rarely uses, or to replace freestanding pieces with fitted units – for example, replacing a wardrobe and chest of drawers in a child's bedroom with a wall-to-wall built-in system, so getting rid of any sharp edges.

Exactly how you change your present home environment, if at all, is your choice and will obviously depend on how much space you have and how much you want to spend. However, we would suggest that next time you buy something new you take your child's safety into account when considering its design.

We have been told having a bath may be dangerous for our son. Is this true?

Possibly, but we cannot say definitely without knowing more about your son's epilepsy (the risks are obviously less for a child whose seizures are either predictable or well-controlled by treatment). A few people with epilepsy do die from drowning each year while taking a bath, but as no specific records of this are kept, we do not know the exact numbers and so cannot put it into proportion. If your son is still young enough to be willing to be supervised while he is having a bath then obviously this would be satisfactory, but with teenagers this is probably unrealistic. If he is insistent on having a bath without direct supervision, then try to make sure that he only bathes when someone else is in the house and that he leaves the bathroom door unlocked. The door should open outwards so that it cannot be blocked if he falls behind it.

A shower would be preferable, as it is safer – it is possible to sustain an injury in a shower, but the chances are far less. Try to avoid shower bases with high surrounding lips, choose a shower fitting with an efficient heat control (ie one which cannot be turned on full accidentally) and make sure that any shower screens are made from safety glass or plastic.

Could our 3-year-old daughter's anti-epileptic drugs be dangerous in overdose?

Yes, and at her young age you should make sure she cannot easily get to her own or any other medication. All drugs should be locked out of the way whenever there is a child in the house (and this includes those that we take for granted such as aspirin and paracetamol). If you do not have a suitable locking cupboard then medicines should be kept at a height which she cannot reach even if she climbs on the furniture.

FINANCE

We have life insurance for our son, which we took out two years ago. Should we tell the company about his recently diagnosed epilepsy? And what if we want to take out other policies for him in the future?

Yes, you should tell the insurance company, since not telling them could invalidate the policy. As your son's epilepsy has been diagnosed well after you took out this insurance, you should have no problems, because the company assessed his risks and set the premiums at the time of writing the policy (ie when it was first taken out).

Most of the major insurance companies will insure people with epilepsy (although some do not) but they may charge extra for doing so. If you have any problems in the future, contact the British Epilepsy Association (address in Appendix 1). Through their brokers they have many types of insurance available for people with epilepsy (including life, accident, motor vehicle and holiday cover) and they should be able to provide a policy for your child.

How the new Disability Discrimination Act will affect insurance provision for people with epilepsy is something that we do not yet know. In theory, the Act will make it against the law for a service provider (and insurance companies are service providers) to make it impossible or unreasonably difficult for anyone to use that service. In practice various exceptions and special conditions will be allowed, so we will just have to wait and see.

Is a child with epilepsy entitled to any sort of disability allowances or benefits?

Not automatically, as it depends on how severe the epilepsy is. As the vast majority of children with epilepsy respond quickly to treatment, most are not entitled to any disability allowances or benefits. The children who may qualify tend to have very frequent seizures and/or another associated condition.

If you think your child may be among those who qualify, you can telephone the Benefits Agency's freephone Benefit Enquiry Line (listed under Benefits Agency in your local phone book) for more information. Your local Citizens' Advice Bureau (again listed in your phone book) may also be able to help, or perhaps one of the epilepsy associations (addresses in Appendix 1). Claiming the correct benefits can be a complicated procedure with many detailed rules to follow, so getting good advice before you start will be invaluable.

If your child is old enough to be going on to higher education, then at some point you will be in contact with your local Education Authority (they will be listed in your local phone book) about the standard maintenance grant. When you speak to them, you could enquire about the additional allowance that is available for disabled students. This extra allowance is related to parental income and is only paid out in very specific circumstances, but if your child has other problems as well as epilepsy then it may be worth asking about it.

Our son has very severe epilepsy and I have to care for him 24 hours a day. Is there any financial help I can get?

You may be able to claim Disability Living Allowance, which is a tax-free benefit for children and adults with disabilities. It has two component parts: the care component which is payable at one of three different rates, and the mobility component payable at two different rates. Each component has a different disability test. The benefit is made payable in the name of the child, not of the parent or carer. If you are successful in claiming either the middle or higher rate care component on behalf of your son, then you should also be able to claim Invalid Care Allowance for yourself, providing that you spend at least 35 hours a week looking after him. Invalid Care Allowance is taxable.

In the answer to the previous question, we said that claiming the correct benefits could be a complicated procedure – now you know why! You are most likely to succeed in your claim if you get advice from people with previous experience of these applications, so don't hesitate to take advantage of their know-how.

Sally will be 16 soon. Will she still be entitled to free prescriptions?

Yes. If she is staying on in full-time education, then all you will need to do is tick the appropriate box on the back of the prescription form and sign it. If she is leaving school at 16 then she will need an exemption certificate.

To obtain an exemption certificate you first need to get a copy of the Department of Health leaflet P11 (called *NHS Prescriptions – How to get them free*) from your doctor, a chemist's or the Department of Social Security. Fill in form B on the leaflet, ask your doctor to sign it and send it off as directed, and in due course Sally will receive an exemption certificate. The actual procedure when you hand in her prescription at the chemist's will hardly change at all – it just means ticking a different box on the back of the form.

Exemption certificates currently last for five years, and Sally will need to renew it at the end of that time by filling in the form again.

CHILDCARE

We are desperate for a night out, but feel uncomfortable about leaving our son with a babysitter. Are we being overcautious?

Not really. You will need to find a babysitter in whom you

have complete confidence and, just as importantly, the babysitter must be confident about managing your son's epilepsy. This should be possible, but you will need to talk things over thoroughly with any potential babysitters, and provide them with all the information they may need (you could base it on the list of information for schools and teachers given in the section on *Teaching the teachers* in Chapter 6). Like any other parents you should make sure that the babysitter knows where you will be and how to contact you easily if there is a problem.

If you know other families with children with epilepsy (perhaps through a local epilepsy group), you could consider coming to some sort of mutual babysitting arrangement with them.

We would like to send our youngest son (who has epilepsy but no other problems) to the same registered childminder who cared for our older two children. She still collects the older ones from school and looks after them until we get home, so we are keen for them all to be together with her. She is happy to do this, so will it be OK, or should we instead look for someone with special training?

Your current childminder should be perfectly capable of looking after your youngest son, providing that you run through all the details of his care with her. You might find the checklist on what to tell a school in the section on *Teaching the teachers* in Chapter 6 useful as a guide for the information she will need.

Speaking more generally, there is no reason why registered childminders should not look after children with epilepsy. The only reason for considering more specialised care would be if a child has other problems as well, and this is discussed in the answer to the next question.

I am a single parent and I have to go out to work to pay the bills. How can I find a childminder who specialises in looking after

children with epilepsy and multiple difficulties like my daughter?

This will not be easy, but there are people who have completed a nursery nursing course (they will have a National Nursery Examination Board qualification, indicated by the letters NNEB) and who take a particular interest in children with special needs. They do not often work independently as childminders – they are more likely to work in special schools or to support children with special needs in mainstream schools. It would be worthwhile trying to find if there is anyone with this type of experience in your area who would be interested in looking after your daughter, perhaps someone who is taking a career break to bring up her own children. You will probably need to use all the contacts and sources of information you have to find them.

If you cannot find a suitable childminder, then you may want to get in touch with your local Social Services department to find out if there are any daycare nurseries for children with special needs in your area. If there are, then they will allocate places on the basis of need, giving priority to parents (and especially single parents like you) who go out to work but who are still on low incomes.

We've been told it might help us get suitable childcare if we had a community care assessment for our daughter. What is this, and would it really be of any help?

All local authorities have the duty to assess the needs of people who require help with daily living (usually because of age or long-term illness or disability) and then, if found necessary, to provide them with suitable support. The assessment process is called a 'community care assessment', and the amount of care provided will depend on the needs of the person being assessed and the resources available locally.

Whether your daughter will be eligible for help will depend on the severity of her epilepsy and if she has any other medical problems. It is unusual for children with epilepsy alone to qualify for any help. However, there is nothing to stop you asking for it! If you get in touch with your local Social Services department they will give you information about requesting an assessment and on the services they can provide.

A community care assessment will not necessarily help you in getting childcare for your daughter – it will depend on what your local authority usually provides. Services available through community care mainly involve practical care in the home, eg you may be offered help in adapting your home to make it safer or more comfortable for your daughter, or they may be able to provide an item of special equipment which she needs. You may also be offered help with holidays for her or with respite care to give you a break (discussed in the answer to the next question).

Our son needs an immense amount of looking after and we are both exhausted. How can we get some sort of break?

The jargon term for this is 'respite care', whether it be a break for a few hours, a whole day, or for long enough for you to have a holiday. Having a break is very important, as you need to be able to recharge your batteries if you are to go on caring for your son. To find out what is available locally, start by contacting your local Social Services department (or ask your son's specialist, who may also be able to offer some advice). The department should arrange for someone to visit you to discuss the particular type of respite care you want, the resources available and any likely cost.

Respite care provision varies considerably from area to area. It may be organised directly by Social Services or by a voluntary agency on their behalf. You may be offered a place in a day centre or day hospital, a residential place in a home, a care attendant to look after your son in your own home, or care in the private homes of families who have registered with Social Services. A useful publication called *Taking a Break* (details in Appendix 3) explains these alternatives, and also discusses the fears and concerns which thoughts of respite care can bring up in carers.

MISCELLANEOUS

What happens if our child has a seizure when he is having dental treatment?

Many parents worry about this. Your dentist should know what to do, but for your own peace of mind it would be preferable to make sure that he or she knows all the details (the type of seizure, the medication your child is taking and any first aid that may be necessary). Tell the dentist about the epilepsy at your child's first appointment after diagnosis.

Dental care and treatment for children with epilepsy can be even more important than usual, because some forms of the drugs (especially the liquid forms) contain sugar which

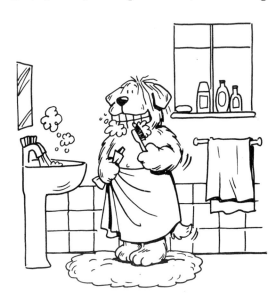

is bad for teeth. Good regular cleaning will usually prevent any problems and liquid medications are now often available as sugar-free preparations. Your child may not like the taste of the sugar-free mixtures and may try to avoid taking them. It is far better to use a medicine containing sugar and to insist on good regular brushing and tooth care than to risk your child missing doses of the sugar-free forms.

Our son is often incontinent when he has seizures in his sleep, and this ruins his bedding. How can we reduce the damage and are we entitled to any financial help?

You can buy waterproof mattress covers, incontinence pads and other forms of protection from a chemist's, but you might like to get some information on what is available before you decide exactly what to purchase. You may have a local Continence Adviser (ask your GP to refer you), or there are various voluntary organisations which can offer advice – try the Continence Foundation's Helpline or the Disabled Living Foundation (all addresses and telephone numbers are in Appendix 2).

Direct financial help to assist with the costs of incontinence is not available, and what other help you can get varies from area to area. In some areas the Social Services department provides a laundry service. Health Authorities have the power to supply aids such as incontinence pads, disposable drawsheets and protective pants free of charge but financial constraints mean that some have decided not to provide such aids at all or to limit the quantity supplied.

Should our son wear or carry some sort of identification saying that he has epilepsy?

This would be a good idea, if you can persuade him to do so. You have a choice of an identity card or a piece of identication jewellery, and they both have their good and bad points.

A number of organisations recommend identity cards as

they can be very useful. They are made of card or plastic and there will be room to write in details of your child's name, address, telephone number, doctor, seizure type and the appropriate first aid. They are available from the various epilepsy associations (addresses in Appendix 1) or your doctor may be able to provide you with one, as some of the pharmaceutical companies issue them free of charge. They have two drawbacks. The first is that people in this country are quite reserved and often will not look through someone's clothes or belongings for such a card. The second is that your son has to remember to take the card with him rather than leave it in the clothes he was wearing the previous day, and he obviously runs the risk of losing it.

Identification bracelets and necklaces are available from three companies – Golden Key, Medic-Alert and SOS Talisman (the addresses are in Appendix 2). Styles vary: on some you would need to have your son's details engraved, while others can be unscrewed to reveal a slip of paper containing the relevant information. Many people think that they are preferable to identity cards as they are far more easily seen, more difficult to lose or forget, and by now most of the population knows that they exist and why. Again they have two drawbacks, the first being that your son may flatly refuse to wear a piece of jewellery! The second is that they can be quite expensive, but if this is a problem you may be able to find a local voluntary organisation to help with the cost. For example, the British Epilepsy Association tells us that in some areas the local Lions Clubs will sponsor identification jewellery for individuals (the Medic-Alert Foundation or your local library should be able to tell you how to make contact with the Lions if there is a club near you).

CHAPTER 8

Travel and holidays

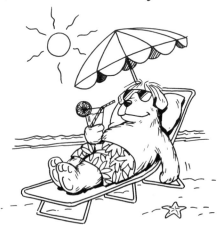

INTRODUCTION

We all enjoy being on holiday, but sometimes the organising needed before we set off is so stressful that we wonder why we are bothering to go at all! When your child has epilepsy, then the list of things you need to remember in your planning becomes a little longer. The suggestions in this chapter are intended to provide practical solutions for these additional concerns.

TRAINS AND BOATS AND PLANES

I've been told that people with epilepsy can obtain a disabled person's railcard. Is this true?

Yes. British Rail have now included people who have continuing seizures as part of this scheme. To apply you will need to complete an application form which should be available from your nearest mainline station. We do not yet know how this scheme will be affected by the current privatisation of the railways, only time will tell.

Is there a similar scheme for bus travel?

At present there is no national scheme, but similar concessionary fare schemes do exist for local bus travel in some parts of the country. Not every area has such a scheme, but where they exist they are organised by local authorities and/or passenger transport executives, and you should contact them for further information (their addresses should be in your local phone book, or your library may be able to tell you how to contact them).

Our daughter hates going by sea. Will the stress of this make her have a seizure while we are on the cross-Channel ferry?

Does your daughter's epilepsy usually become worse when she is under stress? If your answer is that stress can 'trigger' her seizures, then travelling by sea could pose problems. The problem is the stress, not the sailing, so you could start by trying to find out why she dislikes the ferry so much. For example, she may be miserably seasick even in calm weather, in which case it might be worthwhile talking to your GP about a travel-sickness tablet for her (especially as if she is seasick it could affect the efficacy of her antiepileptic drugs). If you cannot discover a cause and work out a solution for it, then you may have to look at other ways of getting to your destination, such as flying or using the Channel Tunnel.

Can flying in an aeroplane bring on a seizure?

For 99% of people with epilepsy it is safe to travel by aeroplane, but a very small number have reported having a seizure during a flight. There is evidence that low atmospheric pressure at very high altitude can make some people's seizures worse, but as the air pressure in an aero-

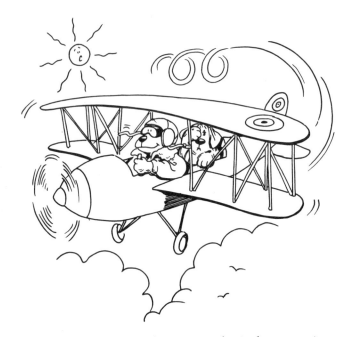

plane is kept constant there is no logical reason (except perhaps stress) why anyone's epilepsy should be worse when flying.

If you are planning a very long flight which involves crossing time zones, you will need to remember that this will affect the timing of your child's medication. It is advisable to adjust the routine gradually over a period of a few days (this also applies to adjusting sleep patterns) rather than making any sudden changes.

Our son has epilepsy and he also uses a wheelchair because of his cerebral palsy. Will airlines be able to accommodate him?

Airlines claim to have a positive attitude to people with special needs, but in practice this is not always obvious. Good planning should help you avoid any potential problems. Make sure the airline knows well in advance about your son's wheelchair, and also about his epilepsy if he still has frequent seizures. They can then arrange for special lifts into the aircraft and allow space so that your access to seating is clear.

ACTIVITIES AND FACILITIES

We are taking our family to a theme park, but it is frightening to think of our youngest son who has epilepsy on some of the rides. Should we let him go on them?

Your son will almost certainly be keen to go on every ride there is, so you will have to talk it over with him and decide exactly what to do. The crucial issues are his type of seizure and their frequency. You have to try and work out the chances of a seizure occurring when he is on a ride and how dangerous this might be – this will depend both on the nature of the ride and his seizure type.

It may help your planning if you can find out full details of the rides before you go. For example, some of these

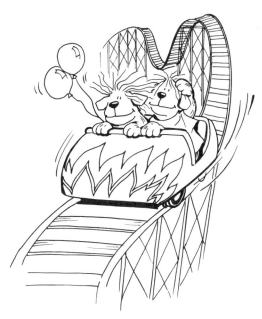

attractions state specifically that people with epilepsy should not use them because they include a flashing light source. Unless your son is photosensitive (this is discussed in the section on *More about seizures* in Chapter 1), this should not be a problem. If you cannot get hold of this information, you will have to establish some basic ground rules with your son and agree to make the final decision on each individual ride when you get there.

Swimming pools in hotels and on camp sites often do not have lifeguards. We do not want to have to tell Sarah that she's not allowed to swim, but what else can we do?

Start by making sure that Sarah is a competent swimmer before you go on holiday (we discuss learning to swim in the section on *Sports* in Chapter 9). It would then be safe to let her swim providing that she always has someone with her to look after her if she does have a seizure. This 'someone' could be you, a friend, or a brother or sister if they are old enough. She should not swim alone, and if the person with her is not a qualified lifeguard then she should keep to shallower water (it should not be deeper than the accompanying person's shoulder height).

Remember that swimming in open water (rivers, lakes or the sea) is more dangerous than in a swimming pool, and so extra precautions should be taken if you decide to allow Sarah to swim in these situations.

Since we booked our holiday, we've been told by a friend that package holiday couriers won't allow children with medical conditions to join in the children's clubs and activity sessions they organise. Is this true?

When you arrive at your hotel or camp site you may have to fill in a form about your child when you arrange for them to join one of these groups. The reaction to you revealing that your child has epilepsy will vary from courier to courier and from holiday company to holiday company and, as usual, will probably depend on whether or not they know anything about epilepsy. Your best approach will be to spend just a few minutes explaining to the couriers about your child's epilepsy and what (if anything) they would need to do if a seizure occurs.

Couriers may be allowed to decide for themselves about whether to allow your child to take part, or they may have to follow the holiday company's policy. For example, they may ask you to sign a disclaimer for any liability if an injury does occur (it is up to you whether or not you sign it). Next time you book a holiday you may like to find out about the company's policy before you spend any money. If you disagree with it, you can explain why and if they will not alter it, tell them you will be taking your custom elsewhere.

We enjoy beach holidays and have usually gone somewhere hot and sunny. This will be our first proper holiday since we were told two years ago that David has epilepsy. Will the heat make his epilepsy worse?

Heat can make epilepsy worse for a small number of children, but if this is true in David's case then you will probably be aware of it already from your experiences here. If there is no evidence that heat affects his epilepsy before you go, then it is unlikely to be affected by the sun while you are away. Remember that too much exposure to the sun is unsafe for other reasons unconnected with epilepsy – it can increase the risk of skin cancer, and children are particularly at risk from sunburn. Like any other child (or adult) David should wear a high protection factor sun cream and keep out of the sun during the hottest part of the day.

Are there hotels that specialise in providing facilities for children like my daughter, who has other medical conditions as well as epilepsy?

There are two national organisations that can provide you with information and advice about holidays for children with special needs like your daughter, including lists of suitable hotels. They are the Holiday Care Service and RADAR (Royal Association for Disability and Rehabilitation), and their addresses are in Appendix 2. They will also be able to advise you about organisations which provide holidays and short breaks away from their parents for children with special needs.

Our daughter wants to go on her school's exchange trip to Germany. What precautions should we think about?

Without knowing more about your daughter – her age, her type of epilepsy and how well she manages it – we can only speak in general terms. Certainly she should be able to go, providing that she knows exactly what to do about her medication and takes an adequate supply of it with her, and that her travel insurance covers her epilepsy (see the next section for more information about these topics). You will also want to check that the teachers supervising the trip know all about her epilepsy and are prepared to be supportive should she need help.

By 'exchange trip', do you mean that your daughter will be staying with a German family? If so, she should make sure that they know about her epilepsy (probably a little information about the appropriate first aid would be enough). If language differences make explanations difficult, then perhaps her teachers could help – we assume that at least one of the teachers accompanying the children will be a fluent German speaker.

The International Bureau for Epilepsy publishes an *Epilepsy Passport* (obtainable through the British Epilepsy Association at the address in Appendix 1). Your daughter might find it useful to take this with her, as it contains information about epilepsy in several different European languages (including German) plus a mini-phrasebook.

Our son leaves school this summer and before he goes to college

in the autumn he wants to travel around Europe with his friends. They are planning to take advantage of those cheap rail tickets for young people and to stay in youth hostels or similar accommodation. How on earth can we stop worrying about him every minute he is away?

Many young people go on this type of trip these days, and all their parents worry about them. After all, it is often the first time that their children have been away from home and unreachable for any length of time. So your own worries are very understandable, and perhaps the best way to deal with them is to reassure yourself that he has planned for any possible problems before he sets off. His choice of transport and accommodation should not cause him any problems, and it should prove to be an exciting and educational experience.

The two essentials are that he has the correct supplies of his medication and the correct travel insurance (both considered in more detail in the next section of this chapter). You will probably also want to check that his friends are confident that they can manage his seizures, should any occur. A copy of the *Epilepsy Passport* (mentioned in the answer to the previous question) might be useful for all of them.

Apart from this, all you can do is what any other parent would do to make sure that their children know how to cope alone abroad. You could try (again like any other parent) to convince him that you would be happier if he rang home regularly to let you know how things were going, and that you would also like to know where they were going and when – but as the essence of this type of holiday is its flexibility, you must not be surprised if you get a call on a different day from a different country!

MEDICAL CARE ABROAD
Will our travel insurance cover Simon's epilepsy?

You should check this before you leave for your holiday, as it is important that he has proper insurance in case he needs medical help while you are away. It is essential that you give details of his epilepsy and any other medical conditions on the insurance application form – they are regarded as 'pre-existing conditions' and if you do not mention them, they will not be covered. If you have any problems getting travel insurance, then contact the British Epilepsy Association (address in Appendix 1) as this is one of the many types of insurance available through their insurance brokers.

We want to go on holiday abroad, but are unsure about emergency medical facilities. Where can we find out more?

From a number of sources – the holiday company, your travel agent, or the British Embassy in the particular country you wish to visit. Any addresses you need should be widely available, perhaps in the tour brochure or from your travel agent. The Department of Health produce a leaflet called the *Traveller's Guide to Health* which you may find useful, and details of how to obtain a copy are in Appendix 3. Once you have the information about your destination, then you will be able to make a sensible decision and, we hope, enjoy an excellent family holiday.

Remember that whatever the level of care available, in many countries you will have to pay some, if not all, of the cost of medical treatment. This means that travel insurance is essential, whether you buy it through your travel agent, your insurance broker or the British Epilepsy Association. Medical attention is free in all European Union countries providing that you have obtained certificate number E111 (from your local Department of Social Security office or Post Office) before you go.

Will our daughter's tablets be available abroad if we need a new supply?

Probably, but it depends where you are going. All the major

anti-epileptic drugs are available in economically-developed parts of the world such as western Europe, the United States and Canada, Australia and New Zealand, and Japan. Their availability elsewhere is much less certain. If she is taking one of the newer drugs such as vigabatrin (Sabril), lamotrigine (Lamictal), gabapentin (Neurontin) or topiramate (Topamax) then you have the additional problem that these drugs are so far only licensed for sale in a small number of countries.

You should also be aware that her tablets may have a different name in another country. The generic name (the true or scientific name of the drug) will be the same but the brand or trade name (the name given to it by the pharmaceutical company that makes it) may not. You can check the names either by contacting the relevant pharmaceutical company or by calling the British Epilepsy Association helpline (phone number in Appendix 1) where they keep a list of the relevant names. At the same time you could ask about the drug's availability at your destination.

If you add on to all this the fact that you will almost certainly have to pay for any drugs you buy abroad (and they can be very expensive), you will see that it is worth taking a good supply of your daughter's tablets with you. In an attempt to avoid any potential problems, it is worth dividing them into two separate packages, keeping one on your person and the other in your hand luggage: suitcases have been known to go astray!

A letter from your doctor stating exactly what has been prescribed for your daughter and why could also be useful, either in case you do need to buy extra supplies or to prevent any difficulties as you go through customs. This letter (which should include the doctor's name and address) may also be of help if a doctor in a foreign country needs more detailed medical information about your daughter's epilepsy and its treatment.

You can also obtain an *Epilepsy Passport* through the

British Epilepsy Association: this not only lists the various European and American trade names of the major antiepileptic drugs, but also has information about epilepsy in several different European languages and a mini-phrasebook.

CHAPTER 9

Your child's social life

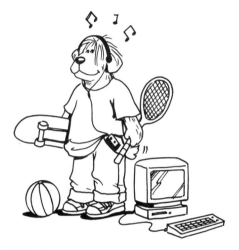

INTRODUCTION

In this chapter we concentrate on those activities children choose to do even though, in practice, children's school and leisure activities often overlap. This overlap means that the advice given here will be equally applicable in school: for example, it will not alter because a computer is being used for class work rather than for playing games, or because sports are being played for a school team rather than a local side. The reverse is also true, and the answers given in Chapter 6 on *School* may prove useful in your child's social life.

The later sections in this chapter concentrate on activities which involve flashing or flickering light. The possible links between disco lighting, computer games, television and epilepsy have received publicity that is out of all proportion to the small scale of the problem that actually exists. You only need to be concerned if your child is photosensitive (this is discussed in more detail in the section on *More about seizures* in Chapter 1) and even then there are ways of preventing problems before they occur.

CLUBS AND ASSOCIATIONS

Will our son be allowed to join the Cubs?

We cannot think of any reason why he should not be allowed to join – and this applies not only to the Cubs, but also to the Scouts, Brownies, Guides and other similar organisations. The information needed by the people running them is very similar to that needed by teachers, and you will find that the general suggestions we give in this answer are discussed in greater detail in the section on *Teaching the teachers* in Chapter 6.

When a child joins one of these organisations you will be asked to complete a medical form. You should mention your son's epilepsy on the form, but you should also see the group's leaders to discuss it in more detail. If they are already knowledgeable about epilepsy, then you will simply need to give them the same sort of information which you will have already given his school. If they know nothing about it, then you will need to start with the basics. If you do come across a negative reaction, it will probably be caused by ignorance, and you should be able to overcome it by providing information about epilepsy and talking about it in a positive way (we make no apologies for our frequent repetitions of this piece of advice!). The various epilepsy associations (addresses in Appendix 1) should be able to help with advice and letters of support if you need them.

Your son should be able to take part in all the organisation's activities, including camp and other visits. If you have particular concerns about anything (for example, your son being away from home), then please discuss them with the leaders to see if a solution can be found.

Our daughter is a keen Guide, and she would like to go on the outdoor pursuits course they are organising. Will she be safe?

All outdoor pursuits courses require stringent safety precautions, and we would hope that these would be enough to keep your daughter safe. However, you do need to take her type of seizure, the severity of her epilepsy (the fewer seizures she has the better) and the particular activities she will be taking part in into account. You (or her Guide leader) should discuss all the facts with the instructors at the centre she will be attending so that they can take extra precautions if they think it necessary. For example, if she goes into status epilepticus (see Chapter 4 for further information about this), then you may need to discuss the use of rectal diazepam (Stesolid) if the trip involves being a long way from hospital care.

Some outdoor pursuits centres now specialise in taking children with multiple difficulties, so it should be possible for your daughter to take part in most activities even if she has other problems as well as epilepsy.

SPORTS

Are there any sports our son should avoid?

The vast majority of sports are perfectly safe for children with epilepsy, providing they are approached sensibly. Your son will need to take all the normal safety precautions required for a particular sport, and then perhaps one or two extra (some of these are discussed in the answers to other questions in this section). However, there are a few less common and higher-risk sports where loss of control due to a seizure could be dangerous even in the best-supervised circumstances: those that spring to mind are scuba diving and motor sports for children such as go-kart racing, and these he should avoid.

The local swimming club won't let our daughter join. Do you think this is fair?

No. It is very important that your daughter learns to swim: she is more likely to drown through being a non-swimmer than by having a seizure in a swimming pool supervised by lifeguards. In a controlled environment like a swimming club, swimming for children with epilepsy is perfectly safe, providing that a few commonsense precautions are taken. If you can explain these to the club, then perhaps they will change their minds about allowing your daughter to join.

Your daughter should never swim alone even if her epilepsy is well controlled – she must have someone with her (perhaps a friend or an older brother or sister) to take care of her should she have a seizure while she is in the water. If she has had seizures within the last two years then it is important that whoever goes with her watches her all the time. Perhaps you could volunteer to go with her to the club if they do not have enough staff to spare someone to keep an eye on her?

The people supervising children's swimming clubs should all be qualified as lifeguards. However, if no qualified lifeguard is available, then your daughter will have to keep to the shallower end of the pool and only swim in water that is no deeper than her companion's shoulder height.

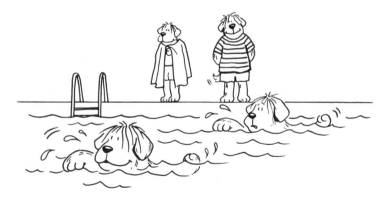

I am worried about our son playing 'mini-rugby' – what if he bangs his head?

Any game of rugby is potentially dangerous, but even so thousands of people enjoy the game every weekend. There are various versions for children, ranging from those in which only touch tackling is permitted up to the full game.

Unless your son's epilepsy was caused by a bad head injury it should be possible and safe, within the regulations of the game, for him to take part. There are specific regulations about the protective equipment that may be worn, but if you are particularly concerned he will probably be allowed to wear a skull cap to protect his head (head collisions are not completely avoidable, even in touch rugby). Perhaps you could talk this through with the person organising your son's team?

We are terrified to let our daughter ride a bike. Are we being overprotective?

Probably not, as most parents these days are frightened when their children start riding bikes, especially when they ride on the road. It is dangerous for any child – with or without epilepsy – to cycle in busy traffic, and caution is required even on less busy side roads. All children should wear protective helmets and brightly coloured clothing when they are out on their bikes.

The best place for your daughter to learn and to continue to ride is somewhere where traffic is restricted. If she still has seizures then it would be preferable for her to keep to grassed areas. As she gets older she will be less willing for you to supervise her, so make sure she knows all the cycling safety rules.

DISCOS

Sean wants to go to his school's end-of-term disco, but a friend has told us that they can cause problems for children with epilepsy. We don't want to forbid him to go unless we have to, but do we have any real choice?

There is a lot of incorrect information around on the subject of discos and epilepsy, and it often leads to unnecessary restrictions being placed on children. There is only one reason why Sean should not go to the disco and enjoy himself, and that is if he is photosensitive (discussed in more detail in the section on *More about seizures* in Chapter 1) AND strobe lighting is to be used (even if he is photo-sensitive he would still be safe providing there were no strobe lights). You could check on the types of lights to be used with the teacher organising the disco.

If a strobe light should be unexpectedly switched on, then Sean could reduce its effects by covering one eye with his hand (closing one eye will not be enough, as light can pass through closed eyelids). This can also be a useful technique for photosensitive children in other situations where flick-ering lights might cause them problems.

But won't the noise at the disco cause problems?

Loud noise, usually heard without warning, can bring on a seizure in an extremely small number of children. Unless you already have evidence of this in your child's case, then the noise at the disco will not be a problem.

TELEVISION

The doctor has told us to make sure our son does not go close to our TV screen. Why?

It sounds as if your son is photosensitive (discussed in more detail in the section on *More about seizures* in Chapter 1), which means that watching television might cause him to have a seizure. The closer he gets to the television, the greater the risk, because the screen with its flickering light will fill more of his field of vision. The flicker is caused by the way television works – the picture is recreated on the screen many times a second.

Your doctor's advice is sensible, but this does not mean that your son needs to stop watching television. With a few sensible precautions he is unlikely to have any additional seizures.

As a rough rule of thumb, he should watch from a distance that is at least four times the size of the screen, ie from at least 2 metres (6–7 feet) for a 48–51 cm (20–21 inch) screen or from at least 2.5 metres (8–9 feet) for a 59 cm (25 inch) model. He should also use a remote control to turn the TV on and off and to change channels.

Turning the brightness control down a little can help, and you may also need to experiment with the lighting in the room where the television is. Some photosensitive children do better watching in a darkened room, while for most others it is better if the room is well-lit.

Is it true that small television screens are better than large ones for children with epilepsy?

Yes, but it only applies to children who are photosensitive. It is usually safer for photosensitive children to watch a small screen, about 40 cms (14 inches) across or smaller, as opposed to anything larger. This is about the size of a small portable television. If you want to check the size of your own set, remember that screen size is measured on the diagonal. They should still watch from a suitable distance, as described in the previous question (for an average small portable this will mean from about 1.5 metres or 5 feet away).

I've heard that wearing sunglasses can help photosensitive children when they are watching television. Does it matter what type of sunglasses they wear?

Sunglasses will not help very much: they will reduce the glare from the screen, but will have no effect on the flicker.

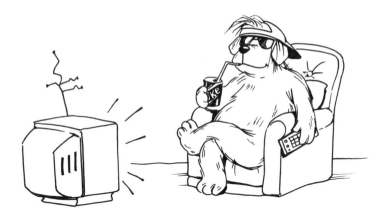

However, you can get special 'television glasses'. The confusion arises because television glasses have polarising lenses, and so do some sunglasses, but the lenses in the television glasses are arranged in a different way from those in the sunglasses.

Television glasses are not used on their own – you also need a polarising filter which fits onto the television screen (the only effect the filter has for people not wearing the glasses is to reduce the screen's glare slightly). The combination of the glasses and the screen mean that the light from the television screen can only reach one eye – and the effects of flicker are reduced if one eye is covered. A photosensitive child could get the same results by covering one eye with a hand or by wearing an eye patch, but the glasses usually prove less inconvenient and more acceptable! The various epilepsy associations (addresses in Appendix 1) should be able to give you details on how to obtain and use them.

Will they ever make televisions that don't affect photosensitive people?

Yes, and in fact they already do. Some televisions now scan the screen at a very fast rate, one which is too fast for the eye to recognise. These 100 Hz televisions are not known to have caused any seizures. You can also buy very small portable televisions which use liquid crystal display (LCD) screens, and these do not flicker at all.

Our daughter watches TV for long periods at a time. Will this be making her epilepsy worse?

It is unlikely to make her epilepsy worse unless she is photosensitive or is excessively tired. Whether it is good for her general wellbeing to turn herself into a couch potato at such a young age is a question we will leave to others to answer! However, you may want to make sure that she is watching TV because she wants to and not because she has lost her confidence about going out (there is a question about this in the section on *Coming to terms with epilepsy* in Chapter 5) or because she is avoiding other children who are teasing her about her epilepsy (teasing is discussed in the section on *Getting on at school* in Chapter 6).

COMPUTERS AND COMPUTER GAMES

My daughter is photosensitive and watching TV is a problem for her. Will using a computer have the same effect?

We all tend to assume that computer monitors and televisions work in the same way – after all, the screen is the same shape and they can both show pictures! However, this is not the case. One of the differences (to be technical for a moment) is that computer monitors flash at a significantly different rate from television screens and also rarely flash at a rate that the human eye can recognise. For example, IBM-compatible machines usually have a flash (reflex) rate of 60 or over per second, a rate which affects very few people, even if they are photosensitive (photosensitivity is discussed in more detail in the section on *More about seizures* in Chapter 1). Most televisions work at a slower rate, and although this is still too rapid for us to be really aware of the flicker, our eyes can still respond to it.

All this simply means that your daughter is unlikely to be affected by using a computer, providing that she is using a proper monitor (if a television is being used as the screen for the computer then that is a different matter, and inadvisable as it could cause some problems). If you are still concerned, then you could consider a computer with a liquid crystal display (LCD) screen which does not flash at all. LCDs are usually found on portable computers, which unfortunately tend to cost considerably more than a desktop model of equivalent power.

Would the filters that you get to fit onto computer screens be of any use?

The filters that you can buy from most computer accessory stores will reduce the glare from the screen, but used alone they have no effect on screen flicker. To reduce flicker you need to combine them with special polarising glasses (the 'television glasses' described in an earlier answer in this chapter). The various epilepsy associations (addresses in Appendix 1) should be able to give you more detailed information about this, and can also advise on suppliers of both the glasses and the filters.

All my son's friends are mad on computer games and although we've stopped him playing them at home because of all the publicity recently, we can't be sure that he's not playing them when he's at their houses. What can we do?

The recent much-publicised scare about a possible link between computer games and epilepsy has led to proper research into the subject being carried out. This research has just been completed and it shows that it is very unlikely that a child would have any additional seizures through playing computer games. If your son didn't have any seizures in the past when you allowed him to play these games at home, and hasn't had any recently when he's been playing secretly in his friends' homes, then he is very unlikely to have them in the future. The advantage of allowing him to play computer games at home is that you will be able to supervise him and make sure that he is being sensible.

If he is photosensitive, then it would be better for him to use a proper computer monitor or one of the hand-held games consoles than to play games on a television screen (if he must use a television screen then he will need to follow the advice given in the section on *Television* earlier in this chapter). You might want to play a few games with him yourself, to see if any of the flashing graphics affect him. It might also be advisable for him not to play when he is very tired.

CHAPTER 10

Growing up

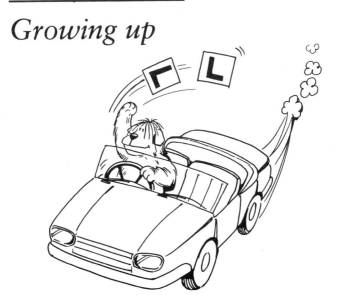

INTRODUCTION

Children with epilepsy are no different from others when it comes to growing up – their preoccupations change from school, computer games and playing with their friends to leaving home, starting work, learning to drive and the possibilities of sexual relationships. Although the emphasis in this chapter is on the practical aspects of these changes and how epilepsy fits into the picture, this does not mean that we have ignored the emotional side. Our aim is to provide you with the information you need to help you deal with your child's changing needs.

DRIVING

Will our daughter be allowed to learn to drive when she is 17?

Yes, if she has had no seizures at all in the last 12 months or has only had seizures in her sleep during the last three years (these times run backwards from the date on which her driving licence takes effect). She must tell the DVLA (the Driver and Vehicle Licensing Agency) about her epilepsy when she applies for her licence. If she contacts the DVLA's Drivers' Medical Unit (address in Appendix 2) they will send her details of exactly what information they need, but basically it is just a matter of completing a form and providing them with the name of her doctor. With her permission, they will then contact the doctor for a medical report that she is fit to drive.

When she passes her test, she will be given a full licence with a limited life, usually for one year at first and then for two periods of three years. Once she has held a full licence and been seizure-free for seven years she will be issued with the standard licence that lasts to the age of 70. If she does have another seizure at any time, whatever the cause and however minor, then she must stop driving and notify the DVLA. Her licence will be withdrawn until she has once again completed the regulation seizure-free period. She will not need to take another driving test to get her licence back.

All these regulations may seem tedious, but the aim is to make driving as safe as possible for everyone. A car out of control is a lethal weapon, and serious accidents can occur in a fraction of a second.

You haven't mentioned medication – does she have to have stopped taking her drugs before she learns to drive?

No. It is very important that she continues to take her anti-epileptic drugs as prescribed to prevent a seizure occurring when she gets her licence and is driving.

If she and her doctors decide that she no longer needs her drugs, then it would be a good idea for her to stop driving during the withdrawal period (which will be several weeks or even months) just in case she has a seizure during this time. She is not legally bound to do this, but it would be the most sensible course of action. Should she have a seizure either after her medication is withdrawn or because of some other change in her treatment (eg switching to a different drug), then she will have to stop driving and give up her licence until she has once again been seizure-free for the required time.

If our son passes his driving test will he be able to go on our car insurance? If so, will it cost a lot more?

The answers to both your questions will depend on your insurance company. Most motor insurance companies now offer cover to people with epilepsy, but some (although not all) charge a higher premium. Other factors – such as the type of car you own, the area you live in, your claims history and your son's age – are likely to have far more influence on the price you will have to pay than your son's epilepsy. You will need to shop around for the best deal, but please ignore any insurance brokers who claim that there is no motor insurance for people with epilepsy, as this is simply not true. If you have any problems, then contact the British Epilepsy Association (address in Appendix 1) as they offer motor insurance through their brokers.

John wants to buy a motorbike, but will he be able to get a licence?

The licensing position is the same for motorbikes as for cars (as discussed in the first question in this section) but insurance is another matter. The British Epilepsy Association's motor insurance scheme does not cover motorbikes, and many people with epilepsy have found it difficult to get suitable cover from other companies.

We live on a farm, so can our son drive on our private land even though he is still having seizures?

It is legally possible for someone without a driving licence to drive on private land, so technically the answer to your question is yes – but are you and he willing to take the risk? Have you considered what would happen if he had an accident? Not only would he risk serious injury, but the costs could be considerable, and you would be very unlikely to be covered by your insurance. If you do decide to allow him to drive, then at no time must he go onto a public highway, however small and quiet. He could face a severe fine or even imprisonment for doing so.

Our son's dream has always been to drive a large lorry for a living. Will he be able to do this?

By a large lorry we assume you mean one for which he would need an LGV (Large Goods Vehicle) licence. He will only be able to obtain such a licence if he has been seizure-free AND off medication for 10 years AND a doctor chosen by the DVLA considers him fit to drive. The same regulations apply to PCV (Passenger Carrying Vehicle) licences which allow people to drive buses and coaches. This is quite a recent change in the law and not everyone is aware of it, so if he does qualify please do not let him be put off by incorrect information.

If he cannot yet qualify for an LGV or PCV licence but does hold an ordinary driving licence, then he will be allowed to drive a light goods vehicle. We would suggest that you contact the British Epilepsy Association's helpline (phone number in Appendix 1) for up-to-date information about the vehicle weight limits involved, as the regulations were being altered just as this book went to press.

WORK

Our daughter leaves school this year and is just starting to look for work. She is worried that she will not get a job if she tells a potential employer about her epilepsy, so should she keep it secret? Is she obliged to tell them about it?

As things stand at present, if she is asked about her health on an application form or at an interview and does not disclose that she has epilepsy, then at any time in the future she can be dismissed for not revealing the information. At the moment there is no legal protection for applicants refused a job on account of their health (even if she could discover that that was the real reason), and almost none for employees dismissed because of their health record.

If you think that this is unfair, then we agree with you. In other countries (for example the USA) employers cannot ask such questions at the application stage. If they ask them after offering someone a job, then only an occupational health specialist (and not the employer) is allowed to make the decision as to whether that person is medically fit for the position. Such a system is far fairer than the current situation in this country, where decisions about fitness for employment are made by people without appropriate qualifications – an arrangement which often leads to unnecessary discrimination.

The new Disability Discrimination Act should, in theory, prevent discrimination in employment. How it will work in practice we do not yet know, and even if it proves effective,

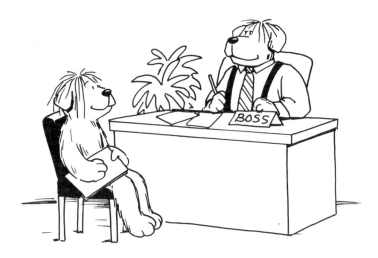

discrimination will still be allowed if the employer can show 'good reason' for it (whatever that may mean). Companies employing fewer than 20 people are exempt from the provisions of the Act, as are organisations such as the police and the Fire Service.

All this leaves your daughter and other people like her in a difficult position, and we cannot offer an easy answer to her problem. You will need to talk it over with her and decide between yourselves whether she should keep quiet about her epilepsy and risk dismissal at some future time, or if she should tell potential employers about it in a way that convinces them that it will not affect her ability to do the job. We would strongly recommend the latter option.

Why are no employers sympathetic towards people with epilepsy?

Not all employers are unsympathetic. Epilepsy is so common that many people involved in management and staff recruitment have friends or family members who have had seizures, and these employers are unlikely to discriminate against other people with epilepsy. There are also companies and organisations with genuine equal opportunities recruitment policies (unfortunately fewer in number than those who claim to have such policies but somehow never put them into effect). In many ways you have to take pot luck: some employers are sympathetic, some are not and it is virtually impossible to find out which employer is in which group. One way of getting more information about your local companies is to contact the Employment Service (the address will be in your phone book) as they have a scheme that recognises employers who show a positive attitude towards people with medical conditions.

After many interviews, our son has still not been offered a job. Is this because of his epilepsy?

His epilepsy might be the reason, but you should not

automatically assume that this is the case. Today's job market is very competitive, so applicants need very good qualifications and the ability to sell themselves to prospective employers. It may be that your son is not doing himself justice: information of how best to present a cv and coaching in interview skills might be more useful to him than worrying about his epilepsy. However, he will also need to work out the best way of telling prospective employers about his epilepsy, and the knowledge and self-confidence to correct any inaccurate ideas about it that they may have.

Are there any specialist employment advisory services for people with epilepsy?

Yes. If your child is still at school or college, then you should get in touch with your local careers advisory service. Contacting them can be a little confusing now that the service has been privatised, but your child's school or college should be able to tell you what to do. If they cannot help, then ask your local TEC (Training and Enterprise Council) for help, or you may find something listed under 'Careers Service' in your local phone book. Your local library may also be able to help with information. Once you have made contact with the service, you should find that there is someone there who specialises in advising children with medical conditions. It might be a particular individual who deals mainly with such children, but in some areas all the members of staff are now trained to provide this type of advice. Because these people inevitably have to deal with a wide range of medical conditions their knowledge of epilepsy may be limited, but if you approach them early enough they should be able to offer constructive advice.

If your child has already left school or college, then you can approach the Employment Service for advice (the number will be in your phone book). Their local Placing, Assessment and Counselling Team (PACT) will include people who specialise in helping adults with a medical condition find work, as well as disability employment advisers who can offer a wide range of services.

If someone is allowed to drive after one year free of seizures, why are they not allowed to enter professions such as teaching and nursing after the same time span?

In some cases they are: it all depends on the school of nursing or the teacher training institution. Quite a number of people with epilepsy are nurses or teachers, but they have sometimes found it difficult to get through the system. It is currently recommended that people with epilepsy should have been seizure-free for two years before they start teacher training, but some institutions will take a candidate's individual circumstances into account before making a decision about admission to the course. Each school of nursing seems to set its own rules, which can be confusing. If someone is committed to either profession there is no reason for them not to press ahead, but they must realise some people will attempt to put barriers in their way.

We hope that in the future the relevant authorities will change their guidelines and bring them into line with those covering driving licences.

Are any jobs legally barred to people with epilepsy?

Yes, some are. They include occupations where having a seizure could be a genuine safety hazard, for example the armed forces, the Fire Service, driving a train or ambulance, or piloting a commercial aircraft. The various epilepsy associations produce excellent leaflets on employment that explain these restrictions and they can also help with up-to-date information on employment law and regulations, as the entry rules for certain jobs do keep changing (for example, organisations such as the police will now consider employing people with epilepsy whereas in the past they would not).

Is a job that requires a driving licence a sensible career choice for our daughter?

We can only give a general answer to this question, as we do not know the details of your daughter's epilepsy, how well it is controlled and how it will affect her in the future. Medical research shows that the longer epilepsy has been controlled, the less likely it is to return. If your daughter has now been seizure-free for some time (eg for three years or more), then such a job would be a perfectly reasonable choice. If she has only been seizure-free for a year, then (although she will be able to hold a licence) it would be sensible for her to wait a little longer before starting on a career where driving was crucial.

Will Jan find it easier to get a job if she registers as disabled?

The new Disability Discrimination Act will bring registering as disabled for employment purposes to an end, so this option will no longer be open to her. There was in any case little evidence that registering as disabled helped anyone's employment prospects (instead it often seemed to have a negative effect) and most people with epilepsy quite rightly chose not to register.

Our 18-year-old son has been told he is unlikely to get a job, so will he still receive the normal state benefits?

There is a difference between being unlikely to get a job and being considered incapable of working because of disability or severe ill-health, and it is not clear from your question which of these applies to your son. We can give a general answer here, but would also suggest that you obtain more detailed information either from the various epilepsy associations (addresses in Appendix 1) or from the Benefits Agency's freephone Benefit Enquiry Line (listed under Benefits Agency in your local phone book).

In general terms then, if your son is capable of working and is actively seeking work (although unable to find a job) then he is entitled to the usual benefits for the unemployed under the usual conditions. If he is assessed as being incapable of work, then as he has not yet reached his twentieth birthday he should be able to claim Severe Disablement Allowance, a weekly cash benefit paid to people who do not have enough National Insurance contributions to qualify for Incapacity Benefit. As qualifying for some benefits can often bring automatic entitlement to others, it would be well worth you getting specific advice for your son's particular circumstances.

MARRIAGE AND OTHER RELATIONSHIPS

We're in the same position as most parents with teenagers – our son has stopped talking to us about his problems. We're fairly sure that he's got worries to do with his epilepsy, but our attempts to draw him out just result in him walking out of the room. Is there anyone he can talk to?

Unfortunately we cannot offer a straightforward answer to this question, as there are no helplines or similar services specifically for children or teenagers with epilepsy. The best we can suggest is that his doctor or his epilepsy specialist nurse (if he has one) might be able to help, especially if he can see them on his own without you being there. Some GP practices now provide counselling services.

If we extend 'talking to' to include 'writing to', then a penfriend with epilepsy would give him the opportunity to share his concerns with someone of a similar age who has similar problems. He could find one through the penfriends page of *Epilepsy Today*, the magazine of the British Epilepsy Association (address in Appendix 1). These days we are all well aware of the dangers of releasing our names and addresses to complete strangers, which is why the BEA operates a box number system for potential penfriends. A potential penfriend will not have to know your son's identity until you are both quite happy that the replies are genuine and that he has made a suitable choice.

If your son is keen on computers and has access to the Internet, then he could join in one of the various epilepsy discussion and support groups that exist in cyberspace – the fact that he could be completely anonymous there might encourage him to communicate when he refuses to do so in person.

Should our son tell his girlfriend about his epilepsy?

Ideally relationships should be built on trust and honesty. It is possible to keep secrets in a close relationship, but it usually imposes a considerable strain on the people involved. If your son does not discuss his epilepsy with his girlfriend and she suspects that he is keeping secrets from her, then she may feel that he does not trust her or she may begin to doubt his honesty. There is also the possibility that other people who know about his epilepsy may accidentally or deliberately let the cat out of the bag.

We therefore think that it is a good policy to talk about epilepsy at a fairly early stage in a relationship. This does not mean blurting out the information before asking for a first date! We hope that your son has developed enough con-

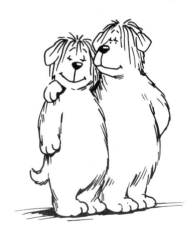

fidence in himself to be able to discuss his epilepsy easily, although we appreciate that it is easier for us to say that than for him to do it. If his girlfriend is truly looking for a serious relationship with him, then revealing that he has epilepsy should not be a great problem. If she is not, then she may make his epilepsy a convenient excuse for breaking things off – in which case he will need reassuring that his epilepsy is not the problem, and that she would have sooner or later found some other reason for ending the relationship.

Our daughter thinks nobody will love her or want to marry her because of her epilepsy. What should we do?

Many people with epilepsy enjoy long and happy marriages or other long-term relationships. Having said that, some research studies have suggested that people with epilepsy are less likely to get married than other people, so your daughter's fears are not entirely unfounded. We do know that people who are confident enough to talk about their epilepsy positively and in context are more successful at developing relationships than those who do not. We hope that the major theme that has been running through this book is the answer: help your daughter to know as much about her epilepsy and herself as possible, so that she can communicate about it with confidence.

From your question it sounds as if your daughter is still thinking negatively about her epilepsy, but she may simply be going through that normal teenage stage of feeling utterly unlovable and unwanted (epilepsy can provide a convenient focus for adolescents who want to put themselves down). Whatever the cause of her lack of self-assurance, the best thing you can do is to encourage her to change her attitude and to be positive about her epilepsy and confident about herself.

Is there any law that will stop our son getting married?

Not in this country. However, this is not true of every

country in the world, so if he is considering getting married abroad he should check first with the relevant embassy.

Our daughter does not want to tell her potential in-laws about her epilepsy. Is this sensible?

It is understandable that she may be apprehensive about this, especially if she does not know them too well. In our opinion she should tell them, preferably when she feels sufficiently comfortable with them to do so. There are some suggestions about how to tell people about epilepsy in the section on *Outside the family* in Chapter 5. We hope the reaction she gets will be positive, but if it is not, then she and her boyfriend will have to work together to educate and reassure his parents, and so in time persuade them to change their attitude.

SEX, CONTRACEPTION AND PREGNANCY

When our son is old enough, will he be able to have normal sexual relationships? Wouldn't sex start up his seizures again?

Yes, he should be able to have sexual relationships that are as 'normal' as anyone else's and no, sex does not trigger seizures. However, in a very few cases anti-epileptic drugs and/or repeated seizures can reduce someone's interest in sex, and then a doctor should be consulted for expert advice.

You do not say if your son has other medical problems as well as epilepsy. If he does, and you are concerned about how his multiple difficulties might affect his sexuality, then we suggest you get help and advice from an organisation called SPOD (Association to aid the Sexual and Personal Relationships of People with a Disability). The address is in Appendix 2.

Will our teenage daughter be able to take the contraceptive pill?

Yes. However, the efficacy of the contraceptive pill is

reduced by some of the major anti-epileptic drugs, for example phenytoin (Epanutin) and carbamazepine (Tegretol, Tegretol Retard). This means a higher-dose pill is needed to provide the same contraceptive effect. Other anti-epileptic drugs have no affect at all on the pill: examples are sodium valproate (Epilim, Epilim Chrono) and the newer drugs such as vigabatrin (Sabril), lamotrigine (Lamictal) and gabapentin (Neurontin).

Most GP practices now have a staff member (either a doctor or a practice nurse) who specialises in providing advice on contraception, and we would suggest that your daughter talks through all the options with them. After all, she might decide that the pill is not for her for reasons totally unconnected with her epilepsy. If she would prefer not to go to the practice (some young women prefer not to see their GPs about contraception), then she could go to a family planning clinic, but she must remember to tell them about her epilepsy and her medication.

Is it possible to have a baby when on anti-epileptic medication?

Most parents of teenage girls probably do not want to think about this question, but their daughters probably do! The answer is yes, and the great majority (about 94%) of women with epilepsy have normal pregnancies and healthy babies. However, there is a risk that the drugs may affect the baby, and we discuss this further in the answer to the next question.

Is anti-epileptic medicine dangerous for the unborn baby?

It can be. None of the anti-epileptic drugs can be considered 100% safe in pregnancy, although some are safer than others. The newer drugs such as lamotrigine (Lamictal) and gabapentin (Neurontin) look safe, but have not yet been in use for long enough for us to be totally sure. It is important to put this risk into context, as the chances of the baby being affected are only slightly higher than average, and most problems caused are minor and can be corrected once the baby is born. However, some drugs in some women will cause more severe harm to some babies, but such problems are extremely rare.

The most dangerous time for the baby is in the first nine weeks of pregnancy, which is why doctors advise women with epilepsy to get expert advice and to plan their pregnancies well in advance so that their treatment can be adjusted if necessary (adjusting or withdrawing treatment can take several weeks or even months). Unfortunately most teenage pregnancies are not planned, and so the danger period has often passed before a young woman has realised she is pregnant. Parents can be reluctant to face up to the fact that their children are sexually active (children have the same feelings about their parents!) but this is not the time for turning a blind eye. If you know or suspect that your daughter is having a sexual relationship, then you should make sure that she gets good advice on contraception now, before it is too late and she becomes pregnant.

Is it very serious to have a seizure during pregnancy?

The vast majority of seizures do not cause any harm to the unborn baby, but it is advisable to try and keep them to a minimum. If a pregnant woman has frequent seizures involving falls or prolonged seizures resulting in a reduced oxygen intake, then there is a slightly increased chance of the baby being harmed in some way. For some women this will mean achieving a careful balance between their medication and their chance of having a seizure – another reason why planned pregnancies are to be preferred.

INDEPENDENT LIVING AND FUTURE CARE

Steve's started to talk about what he's going to do when he's older and goes to college or starts work, gets his own flat and so

on. How can we persuade him that it would be much safer if he stays at home?

You probably can't – it is natural for young people to want their independence. It is just as natural for their parents to worry about them and how they will cope alone. What you can do is to sit down with Steve and work out a compromise between you that gives him the independence he would like, and you the reassurance that he is as safe as possible.

Without knowing more about Steve's epilepsy and his sense of responsibility (which varies widely between individuals and is totally unconnected with epilepsy) then we can only make some general suggestions about what the compromise might be. If his epilepsy is well controlled and he is a fairly mature person, then it would probably be sensible for him to live in a hall of residence or in a shared flat providing that he agrees to take his medication properly. This would give him his independence and you the reassurance that he would not be on his own should he need help. On the other hand, if he has severe problems with his epilepsy or other additional complications, then you might want to investigate the possibility of some form of sheltered housing for him. The various epilepsy associations (addresses in Appendix 1) will be able to help with information and advice.

Talking to our 17-year-old daughter hasn't worked and she is still insisting on leaving home to live with a friend. Isn't there some legislation that will help us make her stay at home?

If your daughter wishes to leave home at her age then there is nothing you can legally do to stop her. We can only suggest that you try discussing your feelings with her again and attempt to come to some sort of compromise which reassures you. If this does not work and she still insists on moving out, then you will have little choice but to try and accept the situation. It will be important to keep the channels of communication open between you, in case she changes her mind and decides that she would prefer to come home until she is a few years older.

Our daughter will never be capable of living alone due to her multiple problems. How should we plan for her future, especially for after our deaths?

You are very wise to be thinking about this now, as it means you can explore all the possibilities and find the solution that bests suits you and your daughter. This is much better than leaving all the decisions until they become urgent. The various epilepsy associations (addresses in Appendix 1) would be good starting points for information.

You should also get in contact with the Social Services department of your local authority. They will be able to tell you about local facilities, and they also have a duty to provide residential care for all those who 'by reason of age, illness, disability or other circumstances are in need of care and attention which is not otherwise available to them'. They will need to make an assessment of your daughter's needs so that they can identify the most appropriate residential placement for her.

You may also be concerned about how the costs of her future care will affect your finances. This is another reason for seeking specialist advice sooner rather than later. The earlier you can start saving, the easier it will be to meet any financial targets you need to set yourself.

Glossary

Terms in *italics* in these definitions refer to other terms in this glossary.

absence seizures *Generalised seizures* involving a brief loss of awareness for several (perhaps 5–20) seconds. They usually occur many times a day, every day, and are often accompanied by eyelid fluttering or lip-smacking or chewing movements.

acupuncture A *complementary therapy* in this country but a traditional form of treatment in China, acupuncture involves inserting special very fine needles into the skin at particular sites on the body in order to balance the 'life energy' or 'vital force' which the Chinese call 'Ch'i' or 'qi'.

AED An abbreviation for *anti-epileptic drug*.

akinetic seizures Derived from the Greek and meaning 'without movement or motion', this is an older and less appropriate name for *atonic* or *astatic seizures*.

ambulatory monitoring A portable type of *EEG* – it literally means 'EEG monitoring while walking about' (from the Latin word 'ambulare' meaning 'to walk'). It allows a child's *brain-waves* to be recorded continuously over anything from several hours to a few days, a much longer time period than is possible with a routine EEG in the out-patients department of a hospital.

anti-convulsant drugs Another name for *anti-epileptic drugs*.

anti-epileptic drugs Drugs used to treat epilepsy, also known as anti-convulsant drugs or AEDs.

aromatherapy A *complementary therapy* involving treatment with essential oils, which are aromatic (scented) oils extracted from the roots, flowers or leaves of plants by distillation.

Aromatherapy often involves massage, but the oils can also be inhaled or added to baths.

astatic seizures Another name for *atonic seizures*.

ataxia Jerky, clumsy, unco-ordinated movements.

atonic seizures or **astatic seizures** *Generalised seizures* involving sudden loss of muscle tone (ie sudden relaxation of the muscles) resulting in a fall. An atonic seizure usually lasts for a few seconds, and may be preceded by a very brief *myoclonic seizure*. 'Atonic' and 'astatic' both come from the Greek: 'atonic' means 'without tone or strength', while 'astatic' means 'unstable' or 'unable to stand'.

attack Another name for a *seizure*.

aura A strange sensation, feeling, smell or taste that acts as a warning that a *seizure* is about to happen. The word 'aura' comes from the Latin and literally means 'breeze'. Not everyone experiences an aura as part of a seizure – people who do usually have *tonic-clonic seizures* or *complex partial seizures* which start in either the *temporal lobe* or the *frontal lobe*. An aura is actually a brief *simple partial sensory seizure*.

autism Autistic children are unable to respond to other people, are extremely resistant to change of any kind, have difficulty learning to talk or to communicate in other ways, and often have additional behavioural problems.

benign Generally speaking, a condition or illness which is not serious and does not usually have harmful consequences. In describing epilepsy it can mean either that the *seizures* are usually controlled very easily with a single *anti-epileptic drug*, or that the epilepsy usually goes into *spontaneous remission* by late childhood.

benign rolandic epilepsy of childhood Full name for the abbreviation *BREC*.

biofeedback A *complementary therapy* based on the fact that it is easier to learn how to alter some aspect of your physical or mental state (ie to develop conscious control of your body's reactions) if you get some sort of reward each time you manage to make the desired change (the 'feedback' part of the name – 'bio' simply means life).

brain scan A painless and completely harmless way of producing clear and detailed pictures of the brain. The two main types are

CT scans and *MRI*; others are *PET* and *SPECT scans*.

brainstem The lowest part of the brain, lying right underneath the *cerebral hemispheres*. It joins all the other parts of the brain to the *spinal cord*. The brainstem controls breathing and heartbeat, and is involved in the co-ordination of certain activities including swallowing and eye movements.

brainwaves Common name for the tiny electrical signals produced inside the brain.

brand name or **trade name** Most drugs have at least two names: the brand or trade name is the name given to a drug by its manufacturer, and is usually written with a capital first letter. The other name is the *generic name*.

BREC This is the commonly-used abbreviation for benign rolandic epilepsy of childhood, a common epilepsy *syndrome* in children. It usually starts at between 4 and 9 years of age and all children grow out of it by their teenage years. Most of the seizures are *simple partial seizures* involving the face and neck. These seizures may then become *secondary generalised tonic-clonic seizures*. The *EEG* usually shows a characteristic pattern. Some children do not require treatment with an *anti-epileptic drug* because the seizures may be very infrequent. Seizure control is good or excellent in those children who are prescribed anti-epileptic drugs.

catamenial seizures *Seizures* which are caused or made worse by menstruation (periods) are called catamenial seizures (from the Greek word 'katamenios' which means monthly).

CAT scan Another name for a *CT scan*.

cerebellum A part of the brain lying just under the back of the two *cerebral hemispheres*. It is connected to many other areas of the brain and to the *spinal cord*. The cerebellum is involved with the control of movements, and co-ordinates the action of all the different muscles.

cerebral hemispheres The two halves of the *cerebrum*. Each hemisphere consists of four areas called *lobes*. The hemispheres are involved in most of our conscious activities and ways of behaving. The left hemisphere controls everything that happens down the right-hand side of the body, while the right hemisphere controls what happens down the left-hand side.

cerebral palsy A medical condition caused by damage to the brain before, during or soon after birth. People with cerebral palsy have problems and difficulties with movement, posture and muscle function, and with weakness of the limbs. 'Cerebral' comes from the Latin word 'cerebrum' meaning 'brain', and 'palsy' is another word for 'paralysis' meaning 'loss of movement or motion'.

cerebrum The largest part of the brain, divided into halves called *cerebral hemispheres.*

classification Generally speaking, to group related topics together into categories in an organised and logical way. In epilepsy, *seizures, syndromes* and types of epilepsy are classified by where they start in the brain, what is known about their causes, the effects they have, and so on. There is an internationally-agreed system for this, and by following it doctors can ensure that they all know exactly which type of epilepsy is being described. Knowing the correct epilepsy classification also helps doctors to decide on the most suitable treatment.

clinical diagnosis The identification of an illness or medical disorder based on what the doctor observes and is told about the symptoms.

clonic seizures *Generalised seizures* involving repeated and rhythmic contractions of the muscles, causing jerks or twitches of the limbs or the whole body. They usually last for between 30 seconds and 1–2 minutes but sometimes last longer. 'Clonic' comes from the Greek word 'klonos', meaning 'turmoil'.

community care assessment The way in which professional staff from a Social Services department work out which community care services someone needs. Community care services are intended to support people who need help with daily living (perhaps because of long-term illness) and enable them to live as full and independent lives as possible, often in their own homes. The amount of care provided will depend on what is needed and on the resources which are available locally.

complementary therapies Non-medical treatments which may be used in addition to conventional medical treatments. Popular complementary therapies include *acupuncture, aromatherapy* and *homeopathy.* Some of these therapies are available through the NHS, but this is unusual, and depends on individual hospitals and GPs.

complex partial seizures *Partial seizures* during which someone's level of consciousness or awareness is affected – the person having the seizure may lose consciousness, or look confused or dazed, or behave in a strange way.

compliance Following medical advice correctly or taking treatment exactly as prescribed. Research has shown that people who are well-informed about their treatment and the reasons for it are more likely to comply with it than those who have not been given the full details.

computed tomography or **computerised tomography** or **computer assisted tomography** or **computerised axial tomography** Alternative names for a *CT scan*.

convulsion Another name for a *seizure*.

convulsive status epilepticus *Status epilepticus* arising from *tonic-clonic seizures*.

corpus callosum The band of nerve fibres joining the two *cerebral hemispheres* together.

cryptogenic epilepsy Describes epilepsy where a cause is suspected but none can actually be found.

CT scan A type of *brain scan* which uses x-rays to produce images of the brain which are then fed into a computer. The computer reconstructs these images into 'slices' – pictures of cross-sections of the brain. When these pictures are viewed in the correct order, they build up a picture of the whole brain. CT stands for computed or computerised tomography (tomography comes from two Greek words – 'tomos' meaning 'a slice' and 'graphein' meaning 'to draw'). It is also referred to as CAT scanning (computer assisted tomography or computerised axial tomography).

cyanosis When the skin turns a blue colour because there is not enough oxygen in the blood. It comes from the Greek word 'kyanos' which means 'blue'.

déjà vu A French phrase which means 'already seen', this is the 'I've been here before' feeling.

developmental delay When a child's physical, mental, emotional and social skills are not developing as they should.

discharges Out-of-the-ordinary *brainwave* patterns that appear on an *EEG* recording. They show that the electrical signals in the brain are not being sent smoothly and in the correct order. The shapes of the discharges and how frequently they occur during the recording provide information about the *seizure* type.

dominant hemisphere Although both *cerebral hemispheres* are important, one usually does far more work than the other. Whichever does the most work is called the dominant hemisphere. In right-handed people (most of the population), the left hemisphere is dominant; in left-handed people, the right hemisphere is usually the dominant one. The control of speech and language usually lies within the dominant hemisphere.

drop attacks or **drop seizures** Older names for *atonic* or *astatic seizures*.

EEG An EEG is a completely safe and painless test which records and measures the tiny electrical signals produced inside the brain. It provides a picture of the electrical activity inside the brain, whether it be the normal activity that goes on all the time or the 'out of the correct order' activity that occurs during a *seizure*. An EEG recording consists of several lines, and each line is a picture of the electrical activity in a different part of the brain (determined by the placing of the *electrodes*). This means that the EEG can show not only what is happening, but also where in the brain it is happening. EEGs are invaluable tools in the investigation and *classification* of epilepsy, although they are not a substitute for a *clinical diagnosis*. They are used to support a clinical diagnosis of epilepsy, and to help decide what type of seizure is involved.

efficacy The ability to produce an intended result. A description usually applied to drugs and how well they work.

electrodes Small discs placed on a child's head during an *EEG* recording to pick up the *brainwaves* and transfer them to the EEG machine.

encephalitis An infection causing inflammation (swelling) of the brain.

excitatory neurotransmitters Types of *neurotransmitters* which work to cause messages to be sent from one *neuron* to another. They are called excitatory neurotransmitters because they excite or stimulate the neurons.

eyewitness The person who actually saw a child having a *seizure*. Before a diagnosis can be made, a doctor needs to be given a very clear, detailed and accurate account of precisely what happened to a child just before, during and after a seizure. The eyewitness is the person who can provide this very important information.

febrile convulsions or **febrile seizures** Convulsions caused by a high temperature (fever). They can occur in young children during a feverish illness, but are unlikely after a child is 4 years old. Febrile seizures are NOT epilepsy.

fit Another name for a *seizure*.

focal seizures Another name for *simple partial seizures* or *complex partial seizures*.

frontal lobes The areas of the *cerebral hemispheres* involved in the control of our voluntary movements and some aspects of our behaviour and emotions.

generalised seizures These occur when the abnormal electrical activity that causes a *seizure* involves both sides of the brain at once (ie the vast majority of the brain). Generalised seizures can be further divided into six types: *absence seizures*; *atonic* or *astatic seizures*; *clonic seizures*; *myoclonic seizures*; *tonic seizures*; and *tonic-clonic seizures*.

generic name Most drugs have at least two names: the generic name is the scientific name (usually written with a small first letter) and applies to all the versions of that drug, regardless of the manufacturer. The other name is the *brand name*.

genes The 'units' of heredity that determine which characteristics we inherit from our parents.

grand mal A French phrase which means 'great illness', this is an older name for *tonic-clonic seizures*.

habit spasms Another name for *tics*.

hemispheres A shorthand way of referring to the *cerebral hemispheres*.

history Information about, and a description of, what actually happened before, during and after a *seizure*. A full medical history will also include other information about someone's health now and in the past, perhaps even back as far as when they were born.

homeopathy A *complementary therapy* based on the principle that 'like can be cured by like' (the word homeopathy comes from two Greek words that mean 'similar' and 'suffering'). The remedies used contain very dilute amounts of a substance which in larger quantities would produce similar symptoms to the illness being treated. Although there is as yet no scientific evidence for why homeopathy works, it is available through the NHS, although the provision is limited.

hyperventilation Overbreathing – breathing very much harder, very much faster and far more deeply than normal. Children are encouraged to hyperventilate during a routine *EEG* (all they have to do is blow rapidly at a tissue or a toy windmill held in front of them) in order to unmask any abnormal electrical activity in the brain. This technique is particularly useful in diagnosing typical *absence seizures*.

hypnotherapy A *complementary therapy* which uses hypnosis. A person who is hypnotised enters a state of very deep relaxation, during which they are more receptive to suggestions of ways of altering behaviour than they would be in a fully-conscious state. While it is most useful in reinforcing good intentions to change bad habits (eg stopping smoking), it can also be helpful in reducing stress and increasing confidence.

hypsarrhythmia A pattern of *discharges* on an *EEG* recording. The name comes from the Greek words 'hypsi' meaning 'aloft' and 'arhythmos' meaning 'absence of rhythm'. A good translation of hypsarrhythmia is 'mountainous chaos' as the EEG recording is full of jumbled irregular peaks.

ictal During a *seizure*. For example, an ictal *EEG* is one recorded while a seizure is actually taking place. 'Ictal' comes from the Latin word 'ictus', which means a strike or sudden blow (the Latin phrase for an epileptic seizure is 'ictus epilepticus').

idiopathic epilepsy or **primary epilepsy** Describes epilepsy for which no obvious cause can be found. 'Idiopathic' means 'of unknown cause' and comes from two Greek words: 'idios' meaning 'own' and 'pathos' meaning 'suffering'.

incidence The incidence of a medical condition is the number of people developing it for the first time during each year (ie the number of new cases within a year).

infantile spasms Another name for *West syndrome*.

inhibitory neurotransmitters Types of *neurotransmitters* which work to prevent or stop messages being sent from one *neuron* to another. They are called inhibitory neurotransmitters because they inhibit or hold back the messages.

interictal Between *seizures*. For example, an interictal *EEG* is one recorded between seizures. 'Inter' is a Latin word meaning 'between', and 'ictal' comes from another Latin word 'ictus',which means a strike or sudden blow (the Latin phrase for an epileptic seizure is 'ictus epilepticus').

intramuscular Into or within a muscle. Often used to describe an injection.

intravenous Into or within a vein. Often used to describe an injection.

jerk attacks or **jerk seizures** Older names for *myoclonic seizures.*

ketogenic diet A medically supervised diet which is sometimes tried as a treatment for the more difficult-to-control types of epilepsy. 'Ketogenic' comes from two other words: 'keto' from 'ketones', which are natural substances found in the blood and urine, and formed from the metabolism (breakdown in the body) of fats; and 'genic' meaning to produce or make. Thus the diet is literally one which 'makes lots of ketones'. It consists mainly of fat, is not very tasty, and must be kept to very strictly under the supervision of a hospital dietician.

learning difficulties Children with learning difficulties have problems in acquiring the practical and behavioural skills needed to cope with everyday living. Learning difficulties can range from the mild (ie simply being slower than other children of the same age in developing these skills) to the severe (ie being unable to develop enough of these skills ever to allow independent living without considerable daily support from other people).

Lennox-Gastaut syndrome This is an uncommon epilepsy *syndrome* which starts at between 1 and 6 years of age. Many different types of *seizure* may occur, including *tonic, atonic, tonic-clonic* and *myoclonic seizures. Status epilepticus* may also occur. There is a characteristic *EEG* showing a pattern called slow spike and slow wave activity. The seizures in this syndrome are usually resistant to most *anti-epileptic drugs*, and therefore seizure control may be difficult. Children commonly develop moderate or severe *learning difficulties* and usually require special schooling.

lesion A general term for any damage or disease affecting a part of the body.

licence The permit which sets out how, when and for whom a drug should be prescribed.

lobes or **lobes of the cerebrum** The areas which make up the two *cerebral hemispheres.* There are four lobes in each hemisphere:

the *frontal lobes*, the *occipital lobes*, the *parietal lobes* and the *temporal lobes*. Each lobe controls or co-ordinates specific activities or functions of the body.

magnetic resonance imaging Full name for the abbreviation *MRI*.

mannerisms Another name for *tics*.

meningitis An infection causing inflammation (swelling) of the membranes (layers of tissue) that cover the brain and *spinal cord* (these membranes are called the meninges).

monotherapy In epilepsy, the use of only one *anti-epileptic drug* for treatment.

MRI A type of *brain scan* which uses magnetism to produce images of the brain which are then fed into a computer. The computer reconstructs these images into pictures of the brain which are similar to those produced by a *CT scan* but much more detailed. MRI stands for magnetic resonance imaging.

myoclonic seizures *Generalised seizures* involving sudden jerky or shock-like contractions of different muscles anywhere in the body, but usually in the arms or legs. Each myoclonic seizure lasts for a fraction of a second, or for one second at most. 'Myoclonic' is derived from the Greek: 'myo-' means 'to do with muscles and 'clonic' comes from 'klonos', meaning 'turmoil'.

nausea Feeling sick, wanting to vomit.

nerve cells Another name for *neurons*.

neurologist A doctor who specialises in treating conditions affecting the brain and nervous system.

neurons The nerve cells that make up the brain and the nervous system. Neurons are responsible for controlling all the actions and functions of every part of the body – seeing, hearing, talking, walking and even thinking. They are the means by which the brain receives, transmits and interprets messages throughout the body. They work by electricity: tiny electrical signals are sent along the neurons, between the neurons throughout the brain, and then down into the *spinal cord* where they can be relayed to any of the other nerves in the body. The actual electrical signals or messages are in the form of chemicals called *neurotransmitters*.

neurotransmitters Chemicals in the brain and nervous system that relay electrical messages between *neurons* (nerve cells). 'Neuro' means to do with nerve cells and 'transmitters' send or communicate signals or messages. There are many different types of neurotransmitter, including *excitatory neurotransmitters* and *inhibitory neurotransmitters.*

night-time seizures Another name for *nocturnal seizures.*

nocturnal seizures or **night-time seizures** 'Nocturnal' comes from the Latin word 'nocturnus' meaning 'during the night'. Because most people sleep at night, this phrase is used to describe *seizures* that occur during sleep.

non-compliance Refusing, failing or 'forgetting' to follow medical advice or a prescribed course of treatment, for example not taking the correct amount of a drug at the correct time of day. The opposite of *compliance.*

non-convulsive status epilepticus *Status epilepticus* arising from *absence seizures* or *complex partial seizures.*

non-epileptic attacks or **non-epileptic seizures** Alternative terms for *pseudoseizures.*

occipital lobes The areas of the *cerebral hemispheres* involved in vision and our interpretation of what we see.

oral To do with the mouth. For example, oral medication is designed to be taken by mouth and swallowed.

paediatric neurologist A *neurologist* who concentrates on, and works only with children.

paediatrician A doctor who specialises in treating children.

paraesthesia Pins and needles in the arms or legs.

parietal lobes The areas of the *cerebral hemispheres* involved in our perception of touch (feeling) and in control of some of our involuntary movements. They are also involved in skills such as reading, writing and dressing.

partial seizures These occur when the abnormal electrical activity that causes a *seizure* starts in one *cerebral hemisphere* or in one *lobe* of one hemisphere. The sensations felt during a partial seizure are determined by the lobe in which the seizure starts. There are two types of partial seizures, called *simple partial seizures* and *complex partial seizures.*

perioral cyanosis *Cyanosis* noticeable around the lips and mouth. 'Peri' is a Greek word meaning 'around' or 'near', and 'oral' comes from the Latin and means 'to do with the mouth'.

petit mal A French phrase which means 'little illness', this is an older name for *absence seizures* or absence epilepsy.

PET scan A type of *brain scan* which provides information about how the brain is functioning as well as showing its structure. At present its use is limited to a few specialised research centres. PET stands for positron emission tomography.

photosensitive epilepsy A *reflex epilepsy* in which *seizures* can be brought on by lights flashing or flickering at certain frequencies (numbers of times per second), by *strobe* lighting, by flickering television sets and other similar triggers. Photosensitivity means being sensitive or susceptible to flashing or flickering lights ('photo-' comes from the Greek and means 'to do with light').

positron emission tomography Full name for a *PET scan.*

post-ictal After a *seizure.* For example, the post-ictal phase describes the time after a seizure. 'Post' is a Latin word meaning 'after', and 'ictal' comes from another Latin word 'ictus', which means a strike or sudden blow (the Latin phrase for an epileptic seizure is 'ictus epilepticus').

prevalence The proportion of a population with a particular medical condition at any one time.

primary epilepsy Another name for *idiopathic epilepsy.*

prognosis A medical assessment of the outlook, expected outcome or probable future course of an illness or disorder.

pseudoseizures or **pseudo-epileptic seizures** *Seizures* which look like epileptic seizures but are not, and which often have an underlying psychological cause. They are more common in girls than in boys, and also in teenagers rather than in younger children. Non-epileptic seizures or attacks is an alternative term for pseudoseizures, and one which is preferred by many doctors.

rectal To do with the rectum (the back passage, also referred to as the anus).

reflex epilepsies A rare group of epilepsies in which a *seizure* can occur in response to a specific trigger or stimulus. The best-known example is *photosensitive epilepsy.*

repeated jerking attacks or **repeated jerking seizures** Older names for *clonic seizures.*

respite care Any facility or resource which allows those who care for sick, frail, elderly or disabled relatives or friends to have a break from their caring tasks. Respite care may be provided in residential or nursing homes, in the person's own home, or with another family.

Sapphire nurse An epilepsy specialist nurse provided by the British Epilepsy Association.

scan In this book, a shorthand way of referring to a *brain scan*.

secondary epilepsy Another name for *symptomatic epilepsy*.

secondary generalised tonic-clonic seizures or **secondarily generalised tonic-clonic seizures** *Seizures* which start as *partial seizures* but then spread to become *generalised seizures* involving the vast majority of the brain.

sedation EEG An *EEG* recording during which a child who has difficulty lying still is given a sedative to help him or her relax or even go to sleep.

seizures Sudden and uncontrolled episodes of excessive electrical activity in the brain. In epilepsy the fault usually lies in a loss of balance between the different *neurotransmitters*. When this happens the electrical signals between the *neurons* are no longer sent smoothly and in the correct order. Instead they are sent out of order, and this 'out of the correct order' signal then often causes an epileptic seizure. This seizure may take the form of a sudden loss of consciousness, involuntary movements, a change in behaviour or a combination of all of these.

side-effects Almost all drugs affect the body in ways beyond their intended actions. These unwanted 'extra' effects are called side-effects. Side-effects vary in their severity from person to person, and sometimes disappear when a body becomes used to a particular drug.

simple partial seizures *Partial seizures* during which someone's level of consciousness or awareness is not affected: there is no loss of consciousness and the person remains completely aware of what is happening.

simple partial sensory seizures *Simple partial seizures* which involve a change in sensation such as a strange (often unpleasant) smell or taste, or unexplained fear, or a feeling of *déjà vu* (the 'I've been here before' feeling), or even tingling and numbness in the face or an arm. An *aura* is an example of a simple partial sensory seizure.

single photon emission computerised tomography Full name for a *SPECT scan*.

sleep-deprived EEG A specialised type of *EEG* recording. Reducing a child's sleep can cause changes in the electrical signals in the brain (it is rare for it to provoke a seizure). These changes would not be seen in a routine EEG, but when they appear after sleep deprivation they may provide important evidence to support a diagnosis of epilepsy.

slices Pictures of cross-sections of the brain produced by a *brain scan*.

SPECT scan A type of *brain scan* which provides information about how the brain is functioning as well as showing its structure. At present its use is limited to a few specialised centres. SPECT stands for single photon emission computerised tomography.

spike and slow wave A characteristic pattern which often appears in an *EEG* recording of someone with epilepsy. This pattern is usually seen in children with *generalised seizures*.

spinal cord An extension of the brain which runs from the *brainstem* down the back inside the bones of the spine. The spinal cord relays information between the brain and the rest of the body, and also controls many of our reflexes.

split screen EEG Another name for *videotelemetry*.

spontaneous remission When an illness gets better of its own accord, it is said to have gone into spontaneous remission. In epilepsy, this means that *seizures* have stopped or 'gone away' and that *anti-epileptic drugs* are no longer needed. However, spontaneous remission only happens in certain types of epilepsy and it is not easy to predict, or even to know exactly when the epilepsy has 'gone away'.

statement of special educational needs Sometimes abbreviated to 'statement'. Many children have special educational needs, ie for some reason they have difficulty in using the mainstream schools in their area. The reason may be a physical disability, a medical or health problem, *learning difficulties* or it may be something else entirely. The statement is the document that sets out the child's special needs and describes all the help that he or she will require in order to receive a broad and well-balanced education. It is based on an assessment of the child's needs carried out by the local education authority. The statement may recommend providing extra support to allow the child to attend a mainstream school, or it may lead to a recommendation for a special school placement.

status epilepticus The currently internationally-accepted definition of status epilepticus is either (a) any *seizure* lasting for at least 30 minutes or (b) repeated seizures lasting for 30 minutes or longer, from which the person did not regain consciousness between each seizure. Status epilepticus is a Latin phrase which simply means 'in an epileptic condition'. It is always a medical emergency.

stiffening attacks or **stiffening seizures** Older names for *tonic seizures*.

strobe Abbreviation for either stroboscope or strobe lighting (stroboscope is the name for the equipment used to produce strobe lighting). Strobe lighting uses high-intensity (extremely bright) flashing lights: the number of flashes per second can be altered very precisely to make moving objects appear stationary. They are often used in discos and amusement arcades, and sometimes used to produce special effects in theatres.

symptomatic epilepsy or **secondary epilepsy** Describes epilepsy where there is a known cause or for which a cause has been identified.

syndrome A cluster of signs and symptoms occurring together in a non-fortuitous (ie non-random or non-coincidental) manner.

telemetry A shorthand way of referring to *videotelemetry*.

television glasses Special glasses which, when used with a special filter on a television screen, allow children with *photosensitive epilepsy* to watch television without triggering a *seizure*.

temporal lobe epilepsy *Complex partial seizures* starting in the the *temporal lobes* of the brain.

temporal lobes The areas of the *cerebral hemispheres* that control our speech, language and hearing, our feelings of fear and anger, and our bowel and bladder functions. They are also involved in behaviour.

tics Regular and repeated uncontrolled and involuntary movements such as eye-blinking, head-shaking, shoulder-shrugging and finger-tapping. They are also called habit spasms or mannerisms. Tics are NOT epilepsy.

tonic seizures *Generalised seizures* involving sudden stiffness of the limbs or the whole body, leading to a fall, often like a tree being felled. The seizure usually ends after 5–10 seconds. 'Tonic' comes from the Greek word 'tonos', meaning 'tension'.

tonic-clonic seizures *Generalised seizures* involving a *tonic* stage followed by a *clonic* stage, ie sudden stiffness and a fall followed by repeated and rhythmic muscle contractions. Most tonic-clonic seizures last 1–3 minutes.

trade name Another name for *brand name*.

tuberous sclerosis An inherited disorder affecting the skin, the nervous system and other organs in the body, which can give rise to epilepsy amongst other symptoms.

tumour An abnormal swelling that forms when cells in a specific area of the body reproduce and increase in number far more quickly than normal.

turn Another name for a *seizure*.

videotelemetry The literal meaning of 'telemetry' is 'measurement from a distance'. Videotelemetry uses a video camera linked to an *EEG* machine, and this combination allows simultaneous recording of what a child is doing and his or her *brainwaves*. When the videotape is played back, one half of the screen shows the child and the other half the EEG recording (which explains the alternative name for this test – 'split screen EEG'). This means that the clinical evidence (what is actually happening to the child) and the electrical evidence (the EEG recording) can be looked at together.

West syndrome Also known as infantile spasms, and named after a Dr West who, over 150 years ago, described infantile spasms occuring in his own son. Infantile spasms are a particular type of *myoclonic seizure* which usually occur in young children between 3 and 10 months old. The spasms usually occur in clusters, with each cluster consisting of 10–50 spasms or more. The spasms are most often seen when the child wakes up and they may be obvious (affecting the whole body, or the arms and legs) or more subtle (affecting only the head or just the eyelids).

APPENDIX 1

Epilepsy associations and organisations

NATIONAL AND REGIONAL ASSOCIATIONS

British Epilepsy Association
Anstey House
40 Hanover Square
Leeds LS3 1BE
Tel: 0113 243 9393
Fax: 0113 242 8804
Helpline tel: 0800 309030

Belfast regional office:
Graham House
Knockbracken Health Care Park
Saintfield Road
Belfast BT8 8BH
Tel: 01232 799355
Fax: 01232 799076

The British Epilepsy Association aims to provide help and support for everyone with epilepsy, their families and those who care for them. This includes helping to provide epilepsy specialist nurses (called Sapphire Nurses) in some areas of the country.

The National Information Centre provides advice and information on any aspect of epilepsy. Enquiries are dealt with by letter or by telephone on the free Epilepsy Helpline (telephone 0800 309030). Advice is also available at BEA's regional office in Belfast.

A comprehensive range of literature is available (including a quarterly magazine called *Epilepsy Today*), as well as many video titles which you can hire or purchase. Schools' information packs are also available. The BEA organises a national network of self-help groups to provide local contact points for help, information and social events. Among other services, the BEA can help with all types of insurance through its brokers.

Epilepsy Association of Scotland
48 Govan Road
Glasgow G51 1JL
Tel: 0141 427 4911
Provides advice and information, education/lecturing services, literature, self help groups and employment training.

Wales Epilepsy Association
Y Pant Teg
Brynteg
Dolgellau
Gwynedd LL40 1RP
Tel: 01341 423339
Provides advice and information, and has local self help groups.

Mersey Region Epilepsy Association
The Glaxo Centre
Norton Street
Liverpool L3 8LR
Tel: 0151 298 2666
A regional association that provides advice and information, literature, lectures and a network of self help groups in Merseyside and North Wales.

Brainwave – The Irish Epilepsy Association
249 Crumlin Road
Dublin 12
Ireland
Tel: 00 3531 455 7500
Provides for Ireland a similar range of services to those provided by the British Epilepsy Association.

INTERNATIONAL ORGANISATIONS

International Bureau for Epilepsy
PO Box 21
2100 AA Heemstede
The Netherlands
Tel: 00 3123 5291019

The staff (who speak excellent English) will provide details of epilepsy associations throughout the world.

OTHER EPILEPSY ORGANISATIONS

The David Lewis Centre
Mill Lane
Warford
Nr Alderly Edge
Cheshire SK9 7UD
Tel: 01565 872613
Provides assessment, respite care, and long term care and education for children and adults with severe epilepsy and learning difficulties.

National Society for Epilepsy
Chalfont Centre for Epilepsy
Chalfont St Peter
Bucks SL9 0RJ
Tel: 01494 873991
Provides residential care, respite care and assessment for adults with severe epilepsy and learning difficulties. Has a small network of self help groups in the community. Provides training and training packages for health and other professionals, and advice and information on epilepsy (including a wide ranging set of literature and video packages).

Park Hospital for Children
Old Road
Headington
Oxford OX3 7LQ
Tel: 01865 741717
Provides assessment for children with severe epilepsy, often with associated learning difficulties.

St Elizabeth's School
South End
Much Hadham
Hertfordshire SG10 6EW
Tel: 01279 843451
Provides long term care and education for children with severe epilepsy and learning difficulties.

St Piers Lingfield
St Pier's Lane
Lingfield
Surrey RH7 6PW
Tel: 01342 832243
Provides assessment and long term care and education for children and young adults with severe epilepsy and learning difficulties.

Services for People with Epilepsy
Head Office
Quarrier's Village
Bridge of Weir
Renfrewshire PA11 3SX
Tel: 01505 612224
Provides assessment and long term care for adults with epilepsy and learning difficulties.

APPENDIX 2

Other useful organisations

Carers National Association
20-25 Glasshouse Yard
London EC1A 4JS
Tel: 0171 490 8818
Helpline tel: 0171 490 8898
  (1.00 pm – 4.00 pm)

Scotland:
11 Queens Crescent
Glasgow G4 9AS
Tel: 0141 333 9495

Supports all people who have to care for others due to medical or other problems.

Children's Head Injury Trust (CHIT)
c/o Neuroscience Unit
The Radcliffe Infirmary
Woodstock Road
Oxford OX2 6HF
Tel: 01865 224786
Provides information, advice and support for families of children who have suffered a head injury.

Contact a Family
170 Tottenham Court Road
London W1P 0HA
Tel: 0171 383 3555
Fax: 0171 383 0259
Promotes mutual support between families who have children with health difficulties through a network of support groups. Publishes excellent guide covering children's health conditions.

Continence Foundation
2 Doughty Street
London WC1N 2PH
Tel: 0171 404 6875
Helpline tel: 0191 213 0050
   (9.00 am – 6.00 pm Monday–Friday)
For help with problems to do with incontinence.

DIAL UK
Park Lodge
St Catherine's Hospital
Tickhill Road
Doncaster DN4 8QN
Tel: 0130 231 0123
Advice on all aspects of disability.

Disability on the Agenda
FREEPOST
London SE99 7EG
Tel: 0345 622 633 (calls charged at local rates)
Textphone: 0345 622 644 (calls charged at local rates)
For leaflets and up-to-date information on the Disability Discrimination Act.

Disabled Living Foundation
380–384 Harrow Road
London W9 2HU
Tel: 0171 289 6111
Information on equipment for people with special needs.

DVLA (Driver and Vehicle Licensing Agency)
Drivers' Medical Unit
Longview Road
Morriston
Swansea SA99 1TU
For enquiries about driving licences.

Employment Service (National Office)
Moorfoot
Sheffield S1 4PQ
Tel: 01142 753275
Provides information on employment advice for people with health problems.

Golden Key
1 Hare Street
Sheerness
Kent ME12 1AH
Tel: 01795 663403
Medical identification bracelets and necklaces.

Headway (National Head Injuries Association Limited)
7 King Edward Court
King Edward Street
Nottingham NG1 1EW
Tel: 0115 924 0800
Provides support and advice for people who have suffered head injuries.

Health Education Authority
Hamilton House
Mabledon Place
London WC1H 9TX
Tel: 0171 383 3833
Promotion of, and publications and videos on, all aspects of general health (eg healthy eating, sensible drinking, stopping smoking, exercise).

Holiday Care Service
2nd Floor
Imperial Buildings
Victoria Road
Horley
Surrey RH6 7PZ
Tel: 0129 377 4535
Holiday advice for people with special needs.

KIDS
80 Waynflete Square
London W10 6UD
Tel: 0181 969 2817
Provides services for families of children with special needs.

Medic-Alert Foundation
12 Bridge Wharf
156 Caledonian Road
London N1 9UU
Tel: 0171 833 3034
Medical identification bracelets and necklaces.

MENCAP
Mencap National Centre
123 Golden Lane
London EC1Y 0RT
Tel: 0171 454 0454
Provides advice and support for people with learning disabilities, their families and carers through a network of local offices and clubs. Includes the Federation of Gateway Clubs.

National Autistic Society
276 Willesden Lane
London NW2 5RB
Tel: 0181 451 1114
Provides advice and information on autism for families and professionals. Owns and manages a number of schools and adult communities for people with autism.

National Council for Voluntary Organisations (NCVO)
Regent's Wharf
8 All Saints Street
London N1 9RL
Tel: 0171 713 6161
The voice of the voluntary sector. Contact for details of any charities in which you may be interested.

Patients Association
18 Guilford Street
London WC1N 1DT
Tel: 0171 242 3460
Provides advice on patients' rights.

RADAR (Royal Association for Disability and Rehabilitation)
12 City Forum
250 City Road
London EC1V 8AF
Tel: 0171 250 3222
Aims to improve the rights and care of disabled people. Information, advice and publications available on topics such as holidays, mobility, leisure, education and employment.

Royal Society for the Prevention of Accidents (RoSPA)
Edgbaston Park
353 Bristol Road
Birmingham B5 7ST
Tel: 0121 248 2000
Information and advice on safety and accident prevention. Please send a stamped addressed envelope with any queries.

SCOPE (formerly the Spastics Society)
12 Park Crescent
London W1N 4EQ
Helpline tel: 0800 626216
   (11.00 am – 9.00 pm Monday–Friday, 2.00 pm – 6.00 pm weekends)
Provides information and counselling service on cerebral palsy and associated disabilities. Manages a number of schools, education centres, units and residential centres for people with cerebral palsy.

SKILL (National Bureau for Students with Disabilities)
336 Brixton Road
London SW9 7AA
Tel: 0171 274 0565
Information line tel: 0171 978 9890
   (1.30 pm – 4.30 pm Monday–Friday)
Information service for students with disabilities.

SOS Talisman
Talman Ltd
21 Grays Corner
Ley Street
Ilford
Essex IG2 7RQ
Tel: 0181 554 5579
Medical identification bracelets and necklaces.

SPOD (Association to aid the Sexual and Personal Relationships
   of People with a Disability)
286 Camden Road
London N7 0BJ
Tel: 0171 607 8851
Provides information and advice on the problems in sex and
personal relationships which disability can cause.

Tuberous Sclerosis Association
Little Barnsley Farm
Catshill
Bromsgrove
Worcestershire B61 0NQ
Tel: 01527 871898
Organises meetings and conferences for families and profes-
sionals. Provides financial help for families, research and special
clinics.

APPENDIX 3

Useful publications

At the time of writing, all the publications listed here were available. Those available through the British Epilepsy Association (address in Appendix 1) are marked with an asterisk. Check with them, the publishers or your local bookshop for current prices.

ABOUT EPILEPSY

General titles

Epilepsy – A Parent's Guide by Joe McMenamin and Mary O'Connor Bird, published by Brainwave The Irish Epilepsy Association (1993)

Epilepsy: The Facts by Anthony Hopkins and Richard Appleton, published by Oxford University Press (1996)

* The Epilepsy Reference Book by Jolyon Oxley and Jay Smith, published by Faber and Faber (1991)

Living with Epilepsy by David Chadwick and Sue Usiskin, published by Optima (new edition due mid-1997)

Living with Epilepsy: A Guide to Taking Control by Dr Peter Fenwick and Elizabeth Fenwick, published by Bloomsbury (1996)

Publications for children

* Hand in Hand (a compilation of letters written by children with epilepsy) edited by Richard Appleton, published by Hoechst Marion Roussel (1993)

* titles available from the BEA

* The Illustrated Junior Encyclopaedia of Epilepsy edited by Richard Appleton, published by Roby Education Ltd for the Mersey Region Epilepsy Association (1995)
* Independence – Epilepsy in Teenagers by Richard Appleton and David Chadwick, published by Hoechst Marion Roussel (1996)
* New Horizons – A Guide for Young People with Epilepsy, pubished by Ciba in association with the Joint Epilepsy Council of the UK and Ireland (1995)

Magazines

* Epilepsy Today, published quarterly by the British Epilepsy Association
* International Epilepsy News, published quarterly by the International Bureau for Epilepsy (available in the UK through the British Epilepsy Association)

Books for professionals

Epilepsy edited by Anthony Hopkins, Simon Shorvon & Gregory Cascino, published by Chapman and Hall (2nd edition 1995)

Epilepsy in Children edited by Jean Aicardi, published by Raven Press (2nd edition 1994)

Other publications

The various epilepsy associations publish a wide range of leaflets, booklets and videos on epilepsy. Write to them at the addresses in Appendix 1 for further details and a current price list.

PUBLICATIONS ON OTHER TOPICS

HEA Guide to Complementary Medicine and Therapies by Anne Woodham, published by the Health Education Authority (1994)

Special Educational Needs – A Guide for Parents, published by the Department for Education and Employment (single copies in various languages free on request by writing to the DFEE Publications Centre, PO Box 2193, London E15 2EU or by telephoning 0181 533 2000)

* titles available from the BEA

Taking a Break, published by the King's Fund Carers Unit (single copies free to carers available from Taking a Break, Newcastle-upon-Tyne X, NE85 2AQ)

Traveller's Guide to Health, published by the Department of Health (single copies free on request by calling Freefone 0800 555 777)

Index

216

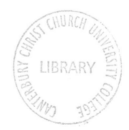

Have you found **Your child's epilepsy: a parent's guide** practical and useful? If so, you may be interested in other books from Class Publishing.

Allergies at your fingertips
Dr Joanne Clough
£11.95 (ISBN 1 872362 52 4)

This comprehensive and practical book covers the complete range of allergies and sensitivities, from minor problems to anaphylaxis, from hayfever to eczema, from diet to environment. It tells you clearly and simply what to do to avoid allergies and how to deal with them when they arise. To be published shortly.

Asthma at your fingertips
NEW REVISED EDITION
Dr Mark Levy, Professor Sean Hilton and Sister Greta Barnes
£11.95 (ISBN 1 872362 06 0)

The more you understand your asthma, the better you can manage it and keep it under good control – and good management makes it easier to live a full, happy and healthy life.

> 'Having asthma should not stop you leading a full and active life ... This book gives you the knowledge. Don't limit yourself.'
> *Adrian Moorehouse MBE, Olympic Gold Medallist*

Diabetes at your fingertips
NEW THIRD EDITION
Professor Peter Sönksen, Dr Charles Fox and Sister Sue Judd
£11.95 (ISBN 1 872362 49 4)

461 questions on diabetes are answered clearly and accurately – the ideal reference book for everyone with diabetes.

> '... you'll find this book a big help.'
> *Gary Mabbutt, England International Footballer*

High blood pressure at your fingertips
Dr Julian Tudor Hart, with a chapter on pregnancy by Professor
Wendy Savage
£11.95 (ISBN 1 872362 48 6)

> 'Readable and comprehensive information for anyone
> with high blood pressure.'
>
> > *Dr Sylvia McLauchlan, Director General,*
> > *The Stroke Association*

Cancer information at your fingertips
Val Speechley and Maxine Rosenfield
£11.95 (ISBN 1 872362 09 5)

> 'I have no hesitation in recommending this book to
> anyone needing more information about cancer. A truly
> useful reference book.'
>
> > *Kay Wright*

Parkinson's at your fingertips
Dr Marie Oxtoby and Professor Adrian Williams
£11.95 (ISBN 1 872362 47 8)

> 'A super DIY manual for patients and carers.'
>
> > *Dr Bernard Dean*

Skin care for psoriasis
Dr V K Dave
£7.95 (ISBN 1 872362 63 X)

> 'Anyone who has psoriasis, or has family members with
> psoriasis, will benefit from reading this easy-to-follow
> practical self-help guide.'
>
> > *Professor C Griffiths, Professor of Dermatology,*
> > *University of Manchester*

PRIORITY ORDER FORM

Cut out or photocopy this form and send it (post free in the UK) to:

Class Publishing   Tel: 01752 202301
FREEPOST (no stamp needed)
London W6 7BR   Fax: 01752 202333

	Please send me urgently (tick boxes below)	**Post included price per copy (UK only)**
☐	**Your child's epilepsy: a parent's guide** (ISBN 1 872362 51 6)	£12.95
☐	**Allergies at your fingertips** (ISBN 1 872362 52 4)	£14.95
☐	**Asthma at your fingertips** (ISBN 1 872362 06 0)	£14.95
☐	**Diabetes at your fingertips** (ISBN 1 872362 49 4)	£14.95
☐	**High blood pressure at your fingertips** (ISBN 1 872362 48 6)	£14.95
☐	**Cancer information at your fingertips** (ISBN 1 872362 09 5)	£14.95
☐	**Parkinson's at your fingertips** (ISBN 1 872362 47 8)	£14.95
☐	**Skin care for psoriasis** (ISBN 1 872362 63 X)	£10.95

TOTAL: _____

Easy ways to pay

Cheque: I enclose a cheque payable to Class Publishing for £_____

Credit card: Please debit my ☐ Access ☐ Visa ☐ Amex
                                        ☐ Switch

Number: _____ Expiry date: _____

My address for delivery is

Name _____

Address _____

Town _____ County _____ Postcode _____

Telephone number in case of query _____

Class Publishing's no quibble guarantee: remember that if, for any reason, you are not satisfied with these books, we will refund all your money, without any questions asked. Prices and VAT rates may be altered for reasons beyond our control.